Hormones in Harmony®

Heal Your Hypothalamus for Optimal Health, Graceful Aging, and Joyous Energy

Deborah Maragopoulos FNP,
The Hormone Queen®

Intuitive Integrative Family Nurse Practitioner blends the Art of Healing with the Science of Medicine to uncover the root of your health problems and help you tap into your innate ability to heal.

*Join The Hormone Reboot Training and Get The Support You Need!:
http://thehormonequeen.genesisgold.com/hnh-hormone-reboot-training

Published by Best Seller Publishing, Pasadena, CA Best Seller Publishing is a registered trademark Printed in the United States of America.

ISBN:9781530964079

Medical Disclaimer:

This book is not meant to be used to diagnose or treat any medical condition.

This publication is designed to provide accurate and authoritative information with regard to the subject matter covered. It is sold with the understanding that the publisher is not engaged in rendering health, medical, or other professional advice. If medical advice or other expert assistance is required, the services of a competent health care professional should be sought. The opinions expressed by the authors in this book are not endorsed by Best Seller Publishing® and are the sole responsibility of the author rendering the opinion.

Most Best Seller Publishing titles are available at special quantity discounts for bulk purchases for sales promotions, premiums, fundraising, and educational use. Special versions or book excerpts can also be created to fit specific needs. For more information, please write:

Best Seller Publishing
1346 Walnut Street, #205
Pasadena, CA 91106
or call 1(626) 765 9750
Toll Free: 1(844) 850-3500

Visit us online at: www.BestSellerPublishing.org

For Mom, whose great love and belief in our healing work will always inspire me

ACKNOWLEDGEMENTS

I want to express my appreciation for everyone who took part in helping me birth this book. My beloved husband Steve who supported me emotionally, physically, and spiritually through the most transformative time of my life. My amazing children Jarys and Kyra who inspire me to share the wisdom I've gained through our life experiences with the world. My awesome assistant Gaby who ran my businesses flawlessly so I was free to write. My dear friend Krisanne who helped me in the editing process. And most of all, my precious Mom who has been with me every step of this healing journey. Thank you, dear ones, I couldn't have done it without you!

TABLE OF CONTENTS

CHAPTER 1

EDUCATE NOT MEDICATE

We all have a story, why we do what we do…

"Daddy, please, don't." My father's stroking my arm. In any other context it would be fine. We are a touchy, feely kind of family. Yet at this moment, I'm in labor with my first child, my senses heightened and every little touch increases my anxiety. I've been in premature labor for the past eleven days.

Ironic, I'm back at my alma mater, UCLA. Last year I graduated from UCLA Nursing School, got married two months later, pregnant five months after that. It's been a rough transformative year. Nana was diagnosed with lung cancer some fifteen months after Poppop died of liver failure. My parents announced their divorce. My husband and I began our new careers. He's a police officer. I'm a nurse. We moved away from our hometown. And now we're having a baby.

It's the first time in my life I've been a patient. First time I've been hospitalized. And I'm really, really sick. Toxemia. That's what they call it. I'm so swollen that the bottom of my feet are round as the bottom of a boat. My toes look like sausages. My blood pressure's super high. I have an outrageous headache. And they're pumping me full of magnesium sulfate to keep me from having seizures. My liver is failing; my kidneys are following suit. My body is rejecting my baby.

And he's trying to come early, some ten weeks early. Yes, he. I had a dream before I conceived that I had a blond, blue-eyed baby boy. I saw him. I held him. My husband and I even named him – Jarys.

Suddenly, I feel a tremendous pressure. The baby is coming! "Daddy, get Mom!"

My father pats my arm reassuringly. "Honey, she's resting. She's been up all night with you."

We've all been up for days. Right now, my husband, Steve, is resting, too, alongside my sisters, his mother, his grandmother. Nana's too sick to be here, but she would if she could. I can feel her holding me some fifty miles away. But even the comfort of her ethereal presence is not enough to take away this awful pressure.

"Go get Mom! The baby's coming!"

"But you said the nurse just checked you…"

She did, just before Dad traded places with Mom. And apparently, I was still only two centimeters. But my baby is premature, really tiny – intrauterine growth retardation – way smaller than he should be at this stage. The pressure nearly brings me out of bed. I know to blow out and not push. Not that I had time to take birthing classes. I went into premature labor and was hospitalized the day before class started. My newly pregnant sister went with Steve to learn the basics in my place. In nursing school, I did a rotation in labor and delivery, this very unit I'm in now. I remember what I taught my patients. But goodness knows, it's easier said than done. I really need to push!

My father runs out of the room to find Mom.

In five more breaths, my short little Italian mother bursts through the curtains, takes one look at my face, peeks under the sheets between my legs, and yells for the nurse!

"Look at me, Deb!" Mom lifts my chin and looks me in the eye. "You can't push. Breathe with me."

"Mom," I gasp between breaths. The contractions are coming faster, harder, right on top of each other. "Steve needs to be here!"

Mom kisses my forehead. "Yes, he'll be with you. Just breathe."

As soon as the nurse arrives and confirms that the baby is crowning, she holds the baby back with one hand, pushes the emergency call light with the other, unlocks the wheels of the gurney with her foot, and maneuvers me out of the room. Mom throws me another kiss and runs, yelling down the hall for my husband.

The next thing I know I'm being prepped for delivery. Steve steps in, dressed in a blue gown, just as the intern doctor gets in position to deliver our baby. My husband looks scared, but so does the intern.

The chief resident steps in, directs the younger doctor to perform an episiotomy to protect our premature baby's head. "But I haven't given her a block."

"There's no time. Do it!"

For the first time since labor began, I cry out in pain. Steve holds me, kissing away my tears, apologizing for the pain that only a woman can know.

And in three heartbeats, out slides Jarys, just as tiny and fair as I saw in my dream. Still I'm surprised at all that blond hair! We're Greek and Italian. Our babies are usually dark.

They whisk my baby away before I can touch him. "Go, Steve, don't let him out of your sight!" He gives me one more kiss. "And whatever you do, only talk to the chief resident!"

I was trained here at UCLA. I know the system well. The "baby docs", the lowest on the MD totem pole, don't know much yet. They're in training. Interns tend to quote the books and not look at the patient. So whatever they say needs to be taken with a grain of salt.

I lie back. I can hear my mother's voice, "What is it? A boy or a girl?" No one answers.

This feels like a dream. I almost died giving birth ten weeks early to a two-pound, seven-ounce baby.

And this adventure has just begun.

The tornado of this birth has carried me into the world of hospitals, doctors, medical research and becoming my child's advocate.

Like Dorothy in the <u>Wizard of Oz</u>, I realize, "We're not in Kansas anymore!"

WHY AREN'T YOU A DOCTOR?

I get asked this question a lot. Especially from patients, after a consult, when I'm the first one to figure out what the root cause of their health problem is, give them a treatment plan, and more so, give them hope that they can achieve optimal health.

"Why aren't you a doctor?"

Well, early on as a premed college student, I volunteered in our local hospital. The nurses seemed to be running the show. And more so, nurses knew how to talk to patients so they could understand what was happening. Plus, all the female doctors I came in contact with were old (granted, I was only eighteen back then) by the time they got married and started to have kids.

The dean was not happy with my decision. "You're at the top of your class. Exceptional in math and hard sciences. You could have your choice of medical schools."

But I wanted it all. Marriage, a family, and a career in health care. So I became a Nurse Practitioner.

It was in nursing school that I really got to appreciate the difference between nursing and medicine. At UCLA, we were taught the bio-psycho-social-spiritual assessment of our patients. We learned that health is a continuum. On one end is optimal wellness, on the opposite end, death.

As a Nurse Practitioner, I look at patients through the lens of wellness, not disease. Physicians study pathophysiology, looking at patients through a disease lens. Conventional medicine tends to focus more attention on treating disease than preventing it and very little attention goes towards trying to optimize health.

Now that's not the fault of physicians. The blame for this Band-Aid level of health care should be placed on the system. Allowing insurance companies to be third party payers gets between the patient and their health care provider. Plus, insurance companies like to dictate treatment protocol and that handcuffs providers. Then you've got the pharmaceutical companies whose bottom line is profit and there's more incentive to keep you sick than heal you.

Spending two weeks of my life in intensive care as a patient changed me as a health care provider. Experience is a great teacher. I was discharged from UCLA Medical Center with greater empathy for my patients. I realized at a very personal level how important communication is between health care providers and patients and their families. And I was bound and determined to go to grad school and become a Family Nurse Practitioner, as soon as possible.

My focus is on optimal health. By the time most patients seek health care, they are already past the midline and heading towards the death side of the health continuum. The first step in helping patients move towards the wellness part of the health continuum is to educate them. And nurses are really good at health education.

Nurse Practitioners are advanced practice nurses, meaning they have higher education and training than the average registered nurse. Nurse Practitioners are licensed to diagnose disease, order and interpret diagnostic tests, and prescribe medications and medical therapies. Different states have different scopes of practice for nurse practitioners but right now in the current health care system, with doctors leaving primary care for specialties, Nurse Practitioners are very much in demand.

I educate rather than medicate.

My goal is to uncover the root of my patients' health issues, provide education regarding their disease and how to reverse it, and then to help them achieve their highest state of wellness – optimal health – body, mind, and soul.

Yes, it's a tall order. But I've doing it for three decades. And I do it well. People come from around the world to consult with me.

Yet I can't help all of them – there's just too many – which is why I wrote this book. Educate the masses and help them realize their potential. That's what I hope for: That by reading this book, you will discover the root of your health issues and how to heal yourself.

Oh, you'll still need health care providers, both conventional and alternative. But with the help of this book, you will be better informed and more likely to partner effectively with your health care provider to achieve your health goals.

SO WHY FOCUS ON HORMONES?

"Oh, my God, Deb!" On the verge of tears, my young husband is beside himself, "I don't know how we're going to afford all the care, the special schools!"

Special schools? Our baby is just hours old! I'm back in intensive care, hooked up to a myriad of IVs, being monitored. Steve's been in the Neonatal Intensive Care Unit watching over our newborn. Reaching over the bedrail, I take his hand. "What is it?"

Barely taking a breath, he cries, "They said our baby will be deaf, blind, and mentally handicapped!"

"What? Who told you this? The intern?" I don't even let him answer. "Does the baby have a rash, like this?" I show him my palm covered in a rash that looks like a blueberry muffin.

He takes my hand. "Oh, no! You have rubella, too!"

"That's impossible! I'm immune so the baby is immune!" This is ridiculous. I need to speak to the chief neonatal resident. "Look, this is a reaction to the antibiotics they gave me. I'm allergic to penicillin. You're allergic to penicillin. Our baby must be, too."

My amniotic sac broke days before they finally let me deliver. That gave them time to give me steroids to try to get the baby's premature lungs to develop. It worked; our baby can breathe on its own.

"There's something else, Deb." Steve leans heavily on the bedrail, exhausted, afraid, looking to me for hope. "They're not sure if our baby is a boy or a girl."

Steve and I meet with the pediatric endocrinologist. Our mothers come with us for moral support. The most renowned pediatric endocrinologist on the West Coast explains that our baby is an XY female, which means the chromosomes are male, but the genitalia appears female.

Because it has androgen insensitivity, she recommends we raise it female. The doctor says, and I quote:

"It's easier to make a hole than a pole."

I'm upset. This doesn't feel right. "But what about our baby's brain? If we raise him as a female and 'she' feels male, let's say by adolescence, then won't 'she' be psychologically confused and possibly damaged by adulthood?"

"We don't know. We only monitor them through childhood. We believe gender identity should match the genitalia and secondary sex characteristics."

I'm just a neophyte nurse sitting in front of a renowned medical specialist, but her logic seems ludicrous. Before I can argue the case of transgender individuals being surgically altered to suit how they feel about their gender identity right here at UCLA, my mother asks, "What's secondary sex characteristics?"

Like a good nurse, I explain the doctor's medical jargon. "She means that if we raise our baby as a boy, he won't have body or facial hair."

Sitting up as tall as her four foot ten-inch frame allows, Mom barks, "That's ridiculous. The child is half Greek and half Italian. The women in our family have mustaches!" Mom's protective energy reminds me of a small dog fending off a bear, "That's no reason to cut off anything!"

So with the support of Mom, I follow my intuition against medical advice and go with our child's DNA, knowing that he may decide later what gender best suited him (or her, or they...)

Our baby was born intersex. Well, at least that's the terminology used today. One in two thousand children are born with ambiguous genitalia. No one knows why.

I know why I gave birth to an intersex child. Jarys is why I do what I do. You see, I had to become a hormone specialist in order to save my child.

And like Dorothy in the <u>Wizard of Oz</u>, I make the best of things. The tornado of birthing an intersex child and then navigating the medical system was a gift. Now it's time to find the Yellow Brick Road.

CHAPTER 2

SICK AND TIRED OF BEING SICK AND TIRED

"I'm sick and tired of being sick and tired!"

My new patient looks sick and tired. Dorothy's got bags under her eyes. Her energy's sluggish and she looks at least ten years older than she claims to be. She came into my office carting a large satchel full of drugs and supplements – everything she's been prescribed or tried on her own over the past few years. Sometimes she gets a bit of relief but nothing lasts. She's seen seven other specialists and no one has been able to help her.

I look at the list of symptoms she's checked off with her comments on my Hormonally Challenged intake form.

- **Fatigue** – need caffeine throughout the day
- **Insomnia** - can't fall asleep or stay asleep
- **No sex drive** – it's ruining my relationship!
- **Irritable** – unreasonable anxiety
- **Depressed** – on meds but not working
- **Brain Fog** – YES! I can't remember anything and it's affecting my job!
- **Changes in Body Fat** – I've put on 20 pounds in the last few years
- **Exercise Intolerance** – I used to be an athlete, but now I'm too tired to exercise
- **Temperature Intolerance** – my feet and hands are cold, but I overheat easily and sweat at night
- **Stress Intolerance** – I can't handle anything anymore.

On the last line, where I ask What's Your Main Concern, she writes:

If I don't get better, I'm going to lose my job, my husband, my life. Please help me!

Dorothy comes to me diagnosed with fibromyalgia and chronic fatigue syndrome. She's on synthetic thyroid hormones, antidepressants, allergy meds. Her cholesterol is elevated, her blood pressure is low, her heart rate is high. Her skin is dry, her hair is thin and brittle, her eyesight is diminished. She complains of frequent bladder and vaginal infections. Her bowels are irregular and she reacts to many foods she used to love. She's tried lots of diets but keeps gaining weight. She's taking so many supplements that it's a wonder she has an appetite for real food.

Dorothy is my typical patient. And Dorothy could be Don. Dorothy is anyone, any age. Dorothy could be you.

You see we're all on a healing path. We're all looking for the Yellow Brick Road that will lead us to optimal health – body, mind and soul.

So let's begin with my new patient Dorothy.

Your hormones affect everything.

Your moods, your memory, your metabolism.

Your appearance, your aging, your appetite.

Your sleep patterns, your stress response, your sex drive.

Everything.

Think of hormones as the software program of the human computer. Many of us are so Hormonally Challenged – sick, aging, tired, or just plain stressed out – that we need a software update.

WHERE EAST MEETS WEST

In my passion for what I want to share with my new patient, I start drawing diagrams to illustrate my points. My patients love them, so much that they take them home, but they're kind of sloppy so I had my artistic daughter draw these for you.

Here's the first one: Where East Meets West

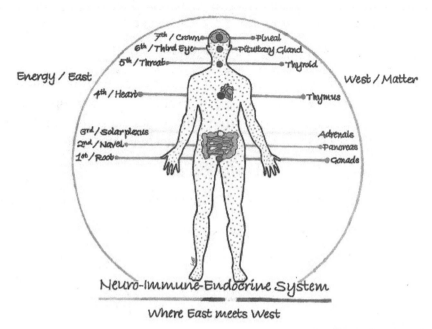

Neuro-Immune-Endocrine System

Where East meets West

There are two philosophies of health care in the world. If you've ever had acupuncture, homeopathy, or body work, then you've experienced energy-based medicine. If you've ever had surgery, taken an antibiotic, or had a cavity filled, then you've experienced matter-based medicine.

Of course energy and matter exist together. Eastern medicine is energy based. Western medicine is matter based. In the West, we assume that if we can't touch it, see it, smell it, it doesn't exist. Yet Einstein proved to us that matter and energy coexist. Matter cannot exist without energy.

If you've ever taken a yoga class, you may have been introduced to chakras. Chakra is a Sanskrit word meaning little wheels of energy. In Eastern medicine, chakras are power points. There are seven chakras. There are seven endocrine glands in your body. Endocrine glands produce hormones. Endocrine glands line up with chakras.

Hormones are the interface between the energy of the environment and the matter of your body. The glands that produce the hormones are the power points.

East meets West in the endocrine system!

Hormones affect everything – our nervous system, our immune system, even digestion and detoxification. These tiny messengers communicate to the DNA within our cells what's happening in the rest of our body as well as what's happening outside in our environment.

Seven chakras. Seven endocrine glands.

- 1st root chakra corresponds with your gonads: ovaries or testes
- 2nd navel chakra corresponds with your pancreas
- 3rd solar plexus chakra corresponds with your adrenal glands
- 4th heart chakra corresponds with your thymus
- 5th throat chakra corresponds with your thyroid
- 6th third eye chakra corresponds with your pituitary gland
- 7th crown chakra corresponds with your pineal gland

From the gonads in the root chakra to the pineal gland in the crown chakra, each gland produces unique hormones that carry energy messages.

Endocrine glands produce hormones. Hormones are messengers. Hormones communicate the energy outside and within your body to the matter of your body – to your cells.

Everything is about communication. If you're running a business and you cannot communicate with your staff, things are going to go wrong.

Same thing in your body. Miscommunication is the basis of dis-ease.

Dis-ease, not disease. Out of balance, out of harmony. Not a permanent state. Dis-ease.

Now when I say hormones, I'm not just talking about sex hormones like estrogen and testosterone. I'm not just talking about thyroid hormones or adrenal hormones. I'm not just talking about insulin or growth hormone or melatonin.

I'm also talking about the hormonal messengers that run your nervous system called neurotransmitters. Neurotransmitters like serotonin and dopamine are just smaller hormones.

And I'm talking about the hormonal messengers that run your immune system called cytokines. You may have heard of interferon or interleukin, these are cytokines, the tiniest of the hormones.

NEURO-IMMUNE-ENDOCRINOLOGY: THE SYMPHONY OF HORMONES

This entire system of hormones is called the neuro-immune-endocrine system. Medicine separates these into three specialties – neurology, immunology, and endocrinology – yet these three systems are dependent upon one another. To truly assess and treat a patient, I take them all into consideration.

While I'm going to focus on your symphony of hormones, your neuro-immune-endocrine system – your biochemistry – is part of the bigger picture that I call:

The DMAR® PYRAMID OF HEALTH

The DMAR® Pyramid of Health is the philosophy that I developed over many years of assessing and treating thousands of patients with hundreds of different complaints. And they all fit into this one system.

The base of the DMAR® Pyramid of Health is ENERGY. Remember, energy is everywhere, energy runs every system, and without energy, matter wouldn't exist. So when I say ENERGY, do I mean electric energy, or magnetic energy, or light energy? Yes, all this and more.

Let's say you walk into a conference room full of people. No one's saying anything, but you feel uncomfortable. You somehow know something's wrong. Perhaps the hair on the back of your neck is standing up, or your gut feels anxious, but you can feel the emotion in the room by its energy.

And guess what, if you're super sensitive, the people don't even need to be there. You could walk in an hour after the angry people left, or a day, or even week later, and feel the energy of their anger.

Have you ever been to a site where many people died? Few people that visit concentration camps can deny that they feel the fear still imprinted in those places. That's energy.

Ok, if this seems a little strange, let me ask the moms how many times have you woken up in the middle of the night knowing something was

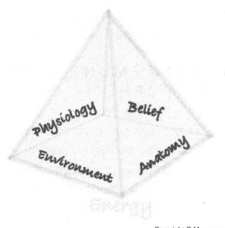

Copyright D Maragopoulos 2016

wrong with your child, rushed to her bedside and found her sick with a fever? That's energy. Your child didn't call out, she's way across the hall, and you were sound asleep. Yet her fear brought you to her side like you were tethered by an invisible cord. It's energy.

ENERGY is the base of the DMAR® PYRAMID OF HEALTH.

A pyramid has four sides.

One side is the **ENVIRONMENT.** Your health is affected by the environment in which you live. If the environment is toxic, your body chemistry is affected. For instance, people who live near nuclear waste, like Three Mile Island, have a higher risk of cancer. We're going to talk about the environment and what you can do to make your environment healthier.

One side is your **ANATOMY.** Your physical structure affects your health. That is the basis behind chiropractic and osteopathic medicine. If you're out of alignment, your health is affected. But it's more than that. I have many patients come to me missing body parts. A woman who's had a hysterectomy does not have the same function as a woman who has her uterus and ovaries intact. Missing body parts, especially endocrine glands, affect how your body functions.

One side is your **PHYSIOLOGY.** The way your body functions is your physiology. Your physiology includes all the biochemical – hormones, neurotransmitters, immune factors, enzymes – that run your physical body. We're going to spend much of this book talking about how to optimize your physiology.

One side is your **BELIEF.** What you believe becomes. That's the basis behind the placebo effect. If you believe enough in a treatment, it'll work, even if that treatment is a sugar pill. And your belief can cause disease. Let me tell you a story about Linda's niece.

Linda came to me with a lump in her genital area. I didn't like the look of it so I biopsied it. It came back as metastatic breast cancer. Only 32 years old, Linda had three young children. Linda's fifteen-year-old niece was very concerned about her own breast health so I examined her. I reassured her that her breasts were healthy, and that she was not at risk of breast cancer like her Aunt Linda. Why? Because Linda's niece was her husband's sister's child. They were not related.

Linda's niece came to see me every month worried about her breast. I counseled her regarding how belief creates reality, trying to teach her visualizations and techniques to release her fear. Yet a few months after Linda died, her niece came to me with a breast mass in the same location of Linda's primary tumor. Her fearful belief created her tumor.

What you believe becomes. And your belief can heal you, too!

YOUR THREE BRAINS

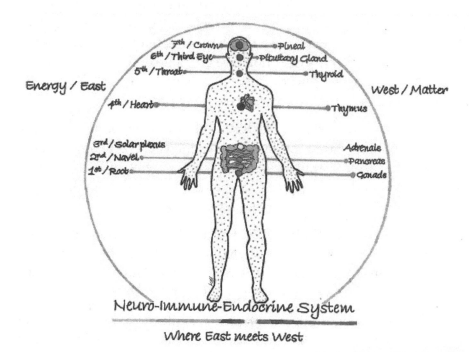

Energy / East

West / Matter

7th / Crown — Pineal
6th / Third Eye — Pituitary Gland
5th / Throat — Thyroid
4th / Heart — Thymus
3rd / Solar plexus — Adrenals
2nd / Navel — Pancreas
1st / Root — Gonads

Neuro-Immune-Endocrine System

Where East meets West

Notice on the East meets West diagram that there are three highlighted areas – one in the head, one in the heart and one in the abdomen. These are your Three Brains. Yes, you have three brains: Your brain, your heart, and your gut. Each of these organs produces the same neurotransmitters.

Neurotransmitters are the hormones of the nervous system. And they're produced by the gut as well as the heart. Ever been nervous before a big event? While your brain fusses over possible outcomes, your heart races and your stomach rumbles. Your heart and your gut make the same neurotransmitters as your brain. In fact, conventional medicine often treats irritable bowel syndrome with antidepressants and everyone knows that you can die of a broken heart (really severe depression means very little serotonin for the heart to function).

And guess what? Your brain is not number one. Nope! Your heart is your number one brain. Your gut is number two. And your brain comes in third. Third in importance. For you can't survive without your heart or your gut, but you can survive without a fully functioning brain. That's why people in comas can survive for years.

Your three brains make up the neuro part of your neuro-immune-endocrine system.

YOUR INTELLIGENT IMMUNE SYSTEM

Now, look at all those little dots on the figure. These represent your white blood cells, the pony express of your immune system. Remember your immune system produces hormones too, called cytokines. Your white blood cells carry the immune messages to all parts of your body.

You know when you're under a lot of stress and you become sick? You catch a common cold virus or break out in cold sores (the herpes virus). Stress affects the adrenal glands which, in turn, affects the immune system.

In the heart chakra lies the thymus – an endocrine gland responsible for programming the white blood cells to know the difference between you and other. Other what? Germs: viruses, bacteria, fungi, even weird cells like cancer. White blood cells (WBC) attack other and spare you. They do so best when you are asleep. Under the influence of melatonin produced by the pineal gland in the crown chakra, the body shuts down normal daytime function and switches into nocturnal mode. The adrenals stop producing the stress hormones adrenaline and cortisol and begin to produce metakephalins that stimulate the thymus to program the WBC's. All hormones, all the time!

High stress means high adrenalin and cortisol production interfering with sleep and effectively turning off the immune system, making you vulnerable to infection and over a very long period of time, cancer.

Your WBCs can travel anywhere in the body, even pass the blood brain barrier delivering messages called cytokines. Cytokines are the tiniest of the "hormones". These minute messengers instigate the immune response, whether that's a breakout of hives in response to an allergen or the attack of an invading virus. The amazing WBC carries on its cell membrane information about all the hormones, all the neurotransmitters, and all the cytokines in the body during its lifetime.

The neuro-immune-endocrine system is a massive communication network that makes the global internet look like child's play.

So if the neuro-immune-endocrine system is the software for the human computer, what's the operating system?

THE OPERATING SYSTEM: YOUR HYPOTHALAMUS

In the center of your brain, your hypothalamus lies vastly unappreciated. Part neurological tissue and part endocrine tissue, your hypothalamus is largely ignored by neurologists as a primitive brain structure. Endocrinologists pay it little heed because they cannot measure its hormones without sacrificing the lab animal. But your hypothalamus is crucial to life.

Your hypothalamus orchestrates your entire symphony of hormones.

If your hormones are harmonious, you are healthy, vital, youthful, and vibrant.

If your hormones are out of harmony, you are sick, tired, aging, stressed, and eventually dis-eased!

So to help the Hormonally Challenged, I focus on the maestro – your **HYPOTHALAMUS**.

CHAPTER 3

Meet the Maestro –
YOUR HYPOTHALAMUS

Alex is hiding behind his mother. She's driven over a hundred miles to have me evaluate and hopefully treat her son. She's one of many parents who have come from all across the state to see me. Mostly they come from the Central Valley bringing children of all ages for me to evaluate.

California is the bread basket of the United States and the Central Valley is filled with toxins – pesticides, heavy metals and petroleum. Every day women conceive in this toxic environment and the result is a high percentage of these children born with developmental disabilities and chromosomal anomalies.

As a parent of a child traumatized by the medical system, I never wear a lab coat. Yet in spite of my child friendly street clothes and my pretty awesome pediatric exam room decorated and filled with toys by my mom, Alex is shy. Evaluated by countless doctors, psychologists and developmental specialists, no one can figure out why this little boy is so delayed. I've seen all his medical records. They can't find anything physically wrong with him, yet Alex has only reached the developmental milestones of a two-year-old. Six years old and Alex has never spoken.

I kneel down at his level. My intuition tells me that Alex's brain is starving. As soon as I think this, Alex peeks from behind his mother's legs. Silently, I tell him, *I'm going to figure out what you need, Alex, so you can wake up.*

Alex emerges from behind the safety of his mother and runs into my arms. He hugs me so tight, I can feel his little body vibrate with gratitude. His mother begins to cry, "He never goes to anyone!"

Three weeks later, Alex speaks for the first time, "Can I go outside and play?"

Overjoyed, his mother calls me right away. "It's working! Alex spoke! The brew is working!"

Brew? What brew?

Let me back up a bit.

Remember, I felt like Alex's brain was starving? Well, my intuition is never wrong. At first I may not understand where it's leading me. My left brain may throw all my medical training, empirical data, and its superior intelligence up in defense, but my intuition is always right. I learned this long ago as a mother, especially as a parent of a sick child, to trust my intuition, and it's served me well in my health care practice.

Now you may also recall that I referred to many parents bringing their developmentally delayed children to me? Small buses of families would come to seek my services. Why? Because when you help one child, the word gets out. These parents were desperate for help. No one was giving them any answers, let alone treatment. Today, these children would probably be diagnosed as autism spectrum disorder. Back in the late nineties, they came to me diagnosed with unknown learning disabilities.

It was the parents that nicknamed my treatment "the brew". You see, back then there was very little available in children's nutritional supplements. Oh, there were some vitamins, but I was formulating a greener "brew", something plant-based, to fill in the nutritional holes in their diets, to make up for the nutrition these children did not receive in their mothers' wombs.

THE HORMONALLY CHALLENGED

People from all over the state and then from all over the country were coming to see me. I already had the reputation of being The Hormone Queen® from years in women's health. Yet when I left conventional medicine to start my own intuitive integrative health care practice, I wanted to learn everything about the neuro-immune-endocrine system. And the universe complied.

Patients with multiple diagnoses, who had been sick for years, came to see me.

Every Hormone issue possible: Thyroid disorders, adrenal disorders, diabetes, growth hormone problems, pituitary failure, menopause, andropause (yes, men go through the change too), PMS, postpartum depression, infertility.

All kinds of Immune disorders: Rheumatoid arthritis, lupus, thyroiditis, colitis, allergies, asthma, dermatitis, cancers of all kinds.

Plus, Neurological disorders: Parkinson's disease, multiple sclerosis, neuropathies, seizure disorders, dementia, depression, anxiety, insomnia, learning disabilities, irritable bowel syndrome (yes, this is neurological and I'll show you why later in the book.)

Most of these patients had multiple problems. I referred to them as Hormonally Challenged.

FAT WHITE MICE AND THE HYPOTHALAMIC CONNECTION

So challenged by the Hormonally Challenged, I began to assess and focus my treatments on the symphony of hormones produced by the neurological, immune, and endocrine systems.

Thanks to some fat white mice, I discovered – rather rediscovered – the **HYPOTHALAMUS.**

I had noticed a triad of disorders in my obese patients. They presented with thyroid disorders, adrenal disorders, and problems with glucose metabolism. On top of all this they were unhappy, oftentimes treated with antidepressants. They wanted relief, preferably something natural. I wanted to figure out what was the common denominator.

What was the root of their issues?

Despite being the late nineties and before fantastic search engines, I diligently researched medical literature and could find nothing. So I focused on animal studies. And that's when I found the fat white mice and **POMC.**

Proopiomelanoncortin or **POMC** is a really, really big hormone produced by the hypothalamus that converts into thyroid releasing hormone **(TRH)**, cortico-releasing hormone **(CRH)**, glucose releasing factor **(GRF)**, melanocyte stimulating hormone **(MSH)**, and beta endorphins. This one hypothalamic hormone controls thyroid function, adrenal function, glucose metabolism, the light sensitivity of your skin and hair, and your state of happiness!

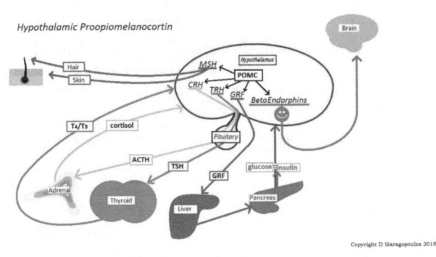

Copyright D Maragopoulos 2016

If one hormone controls all this, what else does your hypothalamus do?

Your Hypothalamus orchestrates:

- Your entire endocrine system – all your hormones
- Your neurological system – all three brains
- Your immune system
- Your weight set point
- Your metabolism
- Your heart and respiratory rate
- Your temperature control
- Your sleep cycles
- Your energy output

- Your sex drive

- Your fertility

- Your skin color

- Your stress response

There's not much that your hypothalamus does not control.

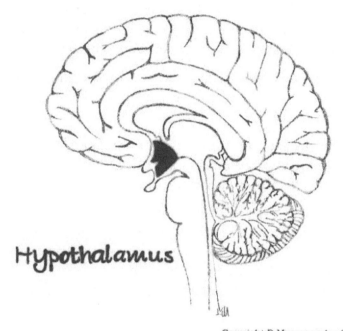

Hypothalamus

Your hypothalamus is the crucial organ in your brain that runs the entire neuro-immune-endocrine system. And when the "hormones" produced by the neuro-immune-endocrine system are out of balance, biochemical miscommunication causes the body to malfunction which leads to dis-ease.

Although we learn about the hypothalamus in premed anatomy and physiology classes, by the time we begin our health care practice, we forget the importance of this primitive brain structure. We just don't appreciate the hypothalamus. We cannot measure the hormones the hypothalamus produces, so we don't deal with it.

Yet the hypothalamus plays a vital role in the orchestration of the symphony of hormones. Hormones sing to your DNA and your DNA dances accordingly. If you're not healthy, you're out of tune. So rather than tune every gland that produces hormones, why not focus on the maestro. Why not balance your Hypothalamus?

FEED YOUR HYPOTHALAMUS

Your brain is protected by a blood-brain barrier. Only glucose and oxygen get through this protective barrier. Your hypothalamus is the only part of your brain that is not protected by this barrier.

Because your hypothalamus is not protected by the blood brain barrier, it is exposed to everything — all nutrients, toxins, pathogens, everything.

Your hypothalamus coordinates all the amino acids that your brain uses to create neurotransmitters. Your hypothalamus filters all the hormones that affect brain chemistry.

In the meantime, I was treating my unhappy overweight patients with nutritional thyroid, adrenal and glucose support, as well as amino acids and bio-identical hormones. Not necessarily sex hormones, but bio-identical thyroid and adrenal hormones, if necessary. I worked with a great pharmacist who could compound anything I dreamt of to help my patients.

Yet I wasn't happy with my treatment regimen. Yes, it was working. Yes, the patients were delighted to be getting better. Yet even though I was giving them natural therapies, I was still creating the same dependency I tried to avoid by not giving them synthetic drugs.

At first I would send my patients out to find the laundry list of supplements. They would come back with the wrong stuff, often with way more than they needed because the health food stores were selling two for one and somebody there convinced them that what they had on the shelf was the same as what I prescribed.

My patients begged me to sell them the nutritional products I was recommending. I didn't want to do it. I wanted to have a pure service-based practice. But their need for the right stuff overcame my defenses, so I researched the best suppliers and started carrying some high quality products.

Yet when I looked at the sheer amount of stuff I was recommending for them to take every day, I thought, could I do it? Like a good nurse, I tried everything I recommended for them. The complexity of their supplement regimens was overwhelming. I couldn't do it, so how could I ask them to take all this stuff?

There had to be a simple and natural way to help their body heal; something to support the hypothalamus, to optimize its function. But what?

PAY ATTENTION TO YOUR DREAMS

"Mom," Fourteen-year-old Jarys rubs my shoulders soothing me after yet another melt down. After months of research, I'm stymied to find something to balance the hypothalamus. And now the computer has crashed again!

"Take a break, Mom. Your energy is affecting the computer." He needs to do his homework and I just messed things up. As if reading my mind, he says, "Don't worry, I'll fix it."

These kids. It's as if their DNA resonates with this new technology. They just get it. I don't.

I get up and kiss him goodnight, then go to tuck in my daughter. Jarys gives me one last piece of advice.

"Why don't you pray about it? Perhaps the answer will come in your dreams."

So I follow my intuitive child's advice and pray to be shown a way to help my patients. I fall asleep asking this question:

What can I feed their hypothalamus to optimize their health – physically, psychologically, and spiritually?

And I have a dream.

I'm standing before a huge tree holding a golden chalice, and my sickest, most Hormonally Challenged patients come and drink from the cup. We never speak, but I know intuitively that they are better. I wake up asking, "What's in the golden chalice?"

And I see, on the screen of my mind, seven letters. They look like Hebrew, but I later discover from a rabbi friend, they're Aramaic.

She has them translated for me, and they are the same seven letters that are the core amino acids in proopiomelanocortin!

Amino acids are designated by single letters. There are twenty-two amino acids that make up all of life. The way amino acids are put together determines the difference between a frog and a cat.

I dream the same dream every night for three months

And every morning I wake up and ask, "What's in the golden chalice?"

The first seven nights, I dreamt the Aramaic letters. Seven sets of seven amino acid combinations.

Starting the eighth night, my dreams revealed even more: Herbs from all over the world, sea vegetation from every sea, ancient sprouted grains, digestive aids, probiotics, adaptogenics, phytonutrients to support detoxification and mitochondrial energy production.

What I had been giving my Hormonally Challenged patients to support their digestion, detoxification, neurological, immune, and endocrine systems, plus so much more. So many bottles of supplements.

Yet my dreams revealed this beautiful synchronistic blend of whole plant foods cradling amino acids designed to support the hypothalamus!

I called it Genesis Gold®.

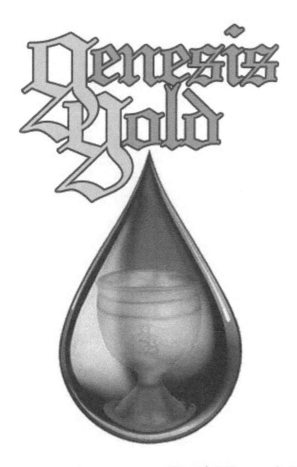

Copyright D Maragopoulos 2016

Finally, I had something to feed my patients to heal them from the inside out.

Genesis Gold® is the foundational formula I was searching for to fill in the micronutrient holes in my patients' diets to optimize their hypothalamus, to balance their hormones, neurotransmitters, and immune function, to improve their digestion and absorption, to optimize their detoxification pathways and energy production.

Genesis Gold® became the Yellow Brick Road that led my patients and me to optimal health.

CHAPTER 4

PLAYING THE HAND YOU'RE DEALT – YOUR DNA

Nicholas was not progressing, still using sign language to communicate at the age of three. His mother was concerned.

I helped deliver Nicholas. His mother was one of my OB patients who followed me to my Intuitive Integrative Health Care practice hoping I could help. Nicholas' mother did everything possible for her son, including giving him special vitamins designed for children like him. Nicholas has Down Syndrome.

Nicholas' doctors thought that his mother's expectations were too high. I believed in her maternal intuition. There was more that could be done to help her son.

"Was he tested for lead?"

His mother shook her head, "No. The pediatrician didn't think it was necessary since we live in a brand new house."

My medical intuition told me that Nicholas' delay was more than his chromosomal anomaly. Something was blocking his cell receptors. I suspected heavy metals. Plus, Nicholas' family lived in an area where food is grown around the freeway. The soil is impregnated by the residue of leaded gasoline. So we tested him for heavy metals.

And his lead levels were off the charts. I treated Nicholas. Just after the first chelation, he began to talk. By the time we were done, Nicholas' speech had surpassed his mother's expectations.

To be safe, I also tested Nicholas' older brother and his parents for lead. Although they lived in the same house, ate the same food, drank the same water, only Nicholas had lead poisoning. Why?

Because the chromosomal anomaly which makes up Down Syndrome affects the detoxification pathways. Nicholas was born with one too many chromosomes. Chromosomes are our genetic material, our DNA. When DNA is damaged, it affects our body's function. That's why Nicholas could not get the lead out of his system and the lead affected the speech center in his brain.

Once we chelated Nicholas, I started him on Genesis Gold® to help him detoxify heavy metals and other toxins he might be exposed to.

YOUR DNA IS NOT SET IN STONE

You might have been taught that you're stuck with the genes you were born with, but that's not true. Your DNA transforms throughout your life.

Most of us were born with one-third of our DNA turned on. That one-third expresses itself in you – the color of your eyes, the freckles on your skin, your bone structure, your keen hearing, your poor eyesight – almost everything about your physical being is expressed by just one-third of your DNA.

Your genotype is your genetic potential. Your phenotype is what your DNA is actively expressing that makes up you. For instance, you can have the genotype for either blue eyes or brown eyes. You have genes for blue eyes from your mother and brown eyes from your father, yet your eyes are green. The color of your eyes is your phenotype. The blue eye genes and brown eye genes are your genotype – your genetic potential.

So if only one-third of your DNA is on, what about the other two-thirds? When the human genome was first opened, genetic scientists called the unexpressed two-thirds of our DNA "junk DNA".

There is no junk. Every single gene has a purpose. We just don't understand it all. But it's not junk. Research has shown that when scientists remove the junk DNA from the fertilized ovum of animals and left the genes known for creating fruit flies, frogs, cats, nothing developed — no larvae, no tadpoles, no kittens. Apparently the unexpressed DNA is not junk. It's needed for life.

So what is it? Well, some of the unexpressed DNA is what was. In your unexpressed DNA is what served your ancestors in the past, like a really long time ago.

During the Ice Age, your ancestors had to hibernate to survive. And in your DNA are the genes for hibernation: Genes that slow down your metabolism so you don't burn energy faster than you can find food to help you survive the longest winter. Genes that make you store fat around your internal organs and form a thick padding around your middle to protect vital organs from the bitter cold. Genes that thicken your blood like antifreeze. Today if those genes are turned on, it's called Type 2 Diabetes.

So are these disease genes? Or are these genes, so vital for survival in the Ice Age when turned on today during global warming, just maladaptive? We don't have disease genes! All our genes are there for a reason. Disease is just maladaptive genetics.

Think of DNA like a deck of cards. You are dealt a certain hand. It may be a good hand. It may be a bad hand. It's all how you play your hand that determines if you win the game. Meaning nature, the DNA you're born with, is influenced by nurture, how you're raised, how you play the game.

Now, some of the unexpressed DNA is what will be, what you might need in the future.

For instance, humans have DNA that is the same as what lizards use to regrow their tails. Wow! What if that got expressed? People who lost limbs might be able to regrow them.

Your DNA is not set in stone. There is so much potential for healing in your DNA. It is always changing.

Remember my first child Jarys? The initial chromosome studies revealed partial androgen insensitivity, meaning his cells were not sensitive enough to testosterone to masculinize. That's why the pediatric endocrinologist told us to raise our child as a girl. It turns out that Jarys did develop secondary sex characteristics – male characteristics. By the time he reached adolescence, his cell receptor sites were no longer resistant to testosterone. His DNA changed.

It's all because of my child that I began to break away from conventional medical thinking. I was trained at UCLA – a very conventional medical center in the 80's. Yet birthing an intersex child transformed my thinking. Anything is possible. Even our DNA can transform.

HORMONES SING & DNA DANCES

Let's focus on your physiology, your biochemistry. I know, I know! Not everyone loves this complicated science like I do, but let me explain.

Physiology is your body's physical function. Anatomy is your body's physical structure. Your physiology is a biochemical soup. I already introduced you to some of your biochemistry — your hormones!

So this side of the DMAR® Pyramid of Health is where your hormones come into play.

Remember, when I say "hormones", I mean your neurotransmitters and immune cytokines, too – the biochemical messengers of the neuro-immune-endocrine system.

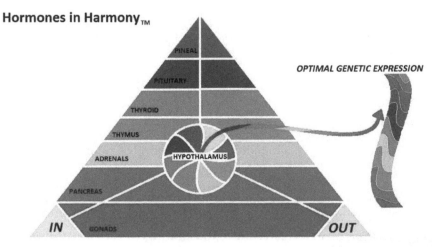

Copyright D Maragopoulos 2016

Do you see how the hormones of the neuro-immune-endocrine system communicate with your DNA?

Your hormones sing and your DNA dances. If your hormones are in harmony, your DNA dances health. If your hormones are out of tune, then your DNA dances like Elaine on Seinfeld – not pretty and not healthy. Your DNA dances dis-ease.

Notice that your Hormones make up most of the pyramid. They're that important! But the entire pyramid is dependent on its base.

The cornerstones of your physiology are **IN** and **OUT.**

IN refers to what you eat and if you digest, absorb, and assimilate your nutrients.

Your hypothalamus is dependent upon your **IN** cornerstone. It needs specific micronutrients to orchestrate the entire neuro-immune-endocrine system. These nutrients become all the hormones, neurotransmitters, and cytokines. This essential nutrition is used to make all your biochemistry like enzymes and electrolytes. What you eat becomes the building blocks for new you.

OUT refers to your detoxification pathways, or how well you clean house. Detoxification includes both liver and kidneys, as well as cellular detoxification. **OUT** also refers to how much energy you produce.

Each of these cornerstones needs specific micronutrients for your body to function optimally.

Very few people get enough essential nutrition from their diets to be perfectly healthy. That's why they need supplementation.

Before I created Genesis Gold®, I was giving my patients lots and lots of supplements to support all the cornerstones of their physiology.

I gave them multiple supplements to support their detoxification pathways and enhance their energy output.

I gave them more supplements to enhance their digestion and improve their absorption of nutrients.

Then I gave them supplements to support their brain chemistry, their immune system, their adrenal glands, their thyroid function, their sex hormones, and more supplements to improve their glucose metabolism.

Yet there was nothing to give them to improve their hypothalamic function.

I know how to eat well. We grow much of our own food. We live in an area that grows organic produce and cage-free, grass-fed, animal protein. We eat fresh seafood, the healthiest fruits and vegetables, the best of what man can gather. Yet it's not enough.

We need to consume that which will optimize our genetic expression. That is why I created Genesis Gold® - to fill in the holes in our diets by providing nutrition from every sea, every continent, encasing the special blend of amino acids necessary to balance your hypothalamus.

Genesis Gold® works by supporting your hypothalamus to keep your Hormones in Harmony®, which means your DNA can express Optimal Health!

CHAPTER 5

IN BETWEEN THE SHEETS

The acrid odor of the mosquito coil fills the hut. The netting over our bed is not enough to deter the insects. Even my husband's protective embrace doesn't protect me. Itchy welts cover my hip. He doesn't have one bite.

Trying not to scratch, I breathe deeply and turn my attention inward. What did I dream last night? The image of a beautiful, perfectly dimpled, olive skinned cherub appears. Almond shaped green eyes with impossibly long lashes like her father, she smiles and a golden energy fills me. I place my hand over my womb.

On the island of Moorea in late summer of 1987, my daughter Kyra was conceived.

Everyone's hormone story begins in their mother's womb.

As a growing fetus, your hormones are higher than they will ever be again. All those hormones help you grow from a tiny zygote to a newborn baby. At birth, you enter a hormonal slump. Although growth occurs, hormones are naturally low in childhood. But at puberty, your hormones are on a fantastic rollercoaster.

First your adrenals start pumping out high levels of DHEA (dehydroepiandrosterone) — the hormone needed to metabolize protein and fat for you to grow rapidly. DHEA converts to testosterone and hair begins sprouting on your body and you develop body odor. DHEA then converts to estrogen. If you have the appropriate receptors, your breasts bud. No estrogen receptors, no breasts.

If you are female, then a couple years later, your ovaries wake up and you have your first first period – menarche.

If you are male, your testes take over the production of testosterone and you begin having wet dreams – nocturnal emissions.

During this time your pancreas pumps out glucagon to release stored sugar in your baby fat and insulin to get that sugar into your cells to fuel your pubescent growth.

For girls it takes a couple years after menarche for growth hormone levels to peak and reach full adult height.

For boys, it's quite a few years later. Sometimes the smallest boys in a high school graduating class end up being the tallest men. They experience their growth spurt in their early twenties.

The earlier you start puberty the sooner you reach your mature adult height. So if you're a small eleven-year-old girl when you get your first period, like my mother was, you may not be very tall.

The last endocrine gland to come to maturity is your thyroid. Thyroid hormone levels reach a plateau to maintain your new young adult basal metabolic rate or BMR.

The Pause follows the same pattern as puberty, but in the opposite direction!

As we came in, thus we go out…

First your adrenals falter. Stress greatly affects you and you get tired easily.

Then your ovaries slow down. Your periods become heavier, irregular, you begin skipping periods. You become moody, irritable, and forgetful. Then fat! Because your pancreas is producing more and more insulin to keep up with the Change and eventually you become insulin resistant.

Men, too, get thick around their middle. They have to work much harder to maintain muscle mass since they're making less testosterone. Some may find a "Dad Bod" sexy, but it's not healthy.

Then growth hormone levels drop and you just don't heal as quickly. You do not recover from exercise or a late night out like you did when you were younger. Finally, your thyroid slows way down. Why? Because you cannot have a high metabolism with low hormones…you would literally implode.

Here's what your hormones look like over your lifetime, thanks to that beautiful baby girl who grew up to be an artistic nurse!

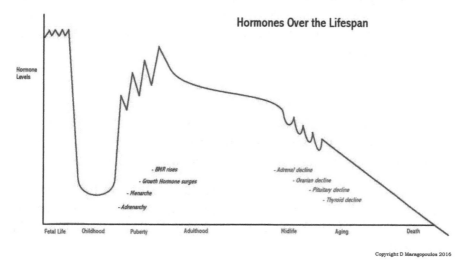

Copyright D Maragopoulos 2016

LET'S TALK ABOUT SEX... HORMONES

Did you know that sex hormones — Progesterone, Testosteronc, Estrogen – are considered steroids? Yep!

Steroids just mean made up of cholesterol. Cholesterol, specifically LDL cholesterol, is the building block for all your sex hormones. That's why when you reach middle age, your cholesterol rises. Your liver is just producing more building blocks for your sex hormones, but your gonads are not using the extra cholesterol to make enough hormones so your LDL cholesterol is high. And not all your LDL, just the large buoyant particles, the safe ones, not the small dense particles that clog up your arteries. That's why I don't treat high cholesterol. I treat your steroid hormonal imbalance.

The difference between the hormones is the size of the molecules.

- Progesterone is the biggest with 21 carbon molecules.

- Testosterone comes in second with 19 carbon molecules.

- And Estrogen is the smallest with only 17 carbon molecules.

Ladies first

I'm going to talk about body parts here, so, men, you may skip ahead to your section below. Right now we're going to focus on the three female sex hormones produced by the ovaries: Estrogen, Progesterone, and Testosterone.

Estrogen is the fertilizer. Estrogen fertilizes the growth of many tissues. Your skin, your hair, your eyes. The lining of your mouth, your gut, your vagina. Your bones, your nerves, your brain. Estrogen helps your tissues grow. But the problem with estrogen is that it fertilizes everything — the roses and the weeds. That's why you need progesterone.

Progesterone is the gardener. Progesterone knows the difference between normal tissue and abnormal growth. Progesterone turns on the cell death gene in tissues that have outlived their welcome, like cancer cells.

Testosterone is the motivator. Testosterone influences your sex drive but more so, testosterone is your mojo – the hormone that pushes you to get ahead, to complete a task, to win. Testosterone motivates you.

Estrogen — the Fertilizer

Estrogens are smallest of the steroids consisting of only 17 carbons. There are three types of estrogen: Estradiol, Estrone and Estriol.

Estradiol: The human ovary produces estradiol (known as E2 because it was discovered after estrone or E1). Estradiol is a powerful growth promoting hormone. It nourishes blood vessels, nerves, skin, hair, nails, and the lining of the gut. Although it does not stimulate new bone formation, estrogen slows the breakdown of existing bone tissue.

Estradiol is the smart hormone. It promotes communication in the brain, enhances memory and creative thinking. As estrogen levels decline, dementia increases.

Estradiol enhances immunity. It stimulates the thymus to promote proper immune programming so that reproductive women produce sufficient antibodies to pass on to their offspring. After menopause, women have a significant decrease in immune function.

Estrone: Since estradiol is short-lived, the body has a backup system of enzymes in the fat cells that can convert estradiol to long-acting estrone. Now there are three main types of estrone — the good, the bad and the ugly.

- The Good = 2OH estrone is the safest form made in great quantities in young women of healthy body weight. The enzyme that promotes 2OH estrone conversion uses the micronutrients found in flax, soy, fatty fish, and cruciferous vegetables (broccoli, cauliflower, cabbage, brussel sprouts).

- The Bad = 4OH estrone, the most volatile of the three, is associated with the most aggressive forms of breast and ovarian cancer.

- The Ugly = 16OH estrone is inflammatory and has been associated with breast and gynecological cancers. Overweight women, sedentary women, women who drink too much alcohol or who have been exposed to xenoestrogens (man-made estrogenic toxins like DDT) and certain drugs like cimetidine make too much of this dangerous estrogen. Fortunately, 16OH estrone can be converted to estriol.

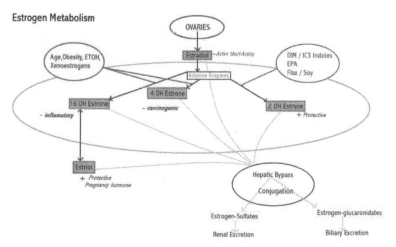

Estrogen Metabolism

Estriol: The dominant hormone in pregnancy is the third estrogen and seems to be the least inflammatory and the most nourishing to vaginal and urethral tissues. Estriol is my favorite bio-identical to use topically to make a dry, atrophic vagina lush.

Progesterone — the Gardener

- Progesterone is the largest steroid hormone, made up of 21 carbon molecules, and produced almost exclusively by the corpus luteum of the ovaries (the little cave left over after the egg of the month ovulates).

- 5% of a woman's progesterone comes from the conversion of pregnenolone in the adrenals. When under stress, the adrenals steal progesterone from the ovaries to make cortisol. That's why your periods can become irregular when you're stressed.

- Progesterone has a calming effect to help with anxiety and insomnia.

- Progesterone, along with testosterone, DHEA and growth hormone, stimulates new bone formation (to fight osteoporosis).

Testosterone – the Motivator

- Testosterone is an androgenic 19 carbon molecule produced by the ovaries.

- There are two menstrual surges of testosterone that mirror estrogen decline – right before ovulation and right before menstruation.

- Male testosterone levels follow their mates' menstrual cycles.

- Testosterone converts into DHT – dihydrotestosterone – which is the active male hormone responsible for male-pattern baldness.

Now, Men, how's your T?

Testosterone is the hormone of manliness. Yes, women make testosterone, too, yet men make much more to achieve the body size, muscle mass, bone density and strength associated with manhood. Low testosterone levels contribute to infertility, loss of lean body mass, increased body fat, moodiness and even hot flashes. Yes, men have hot flashes, too.

Testosterone is falling. Since 1997, when I left women's health for family practice, I've measured hundreds of men's hormones. Nearly twenty years ago the normal ranges were much, much higher. Now they've dropped significantly, especially testosterone levels in men. Are men becoming feminized? Yes!

Stress, lack of exercise, highly processed foods and exposure to xenoestrogens (synthetic chemicals that have estrogenic effects like those found in pesticides and plastics) depletes testosterone levels.

You may be told that your testosterone levels are within normal ranges, but I'll tell you that those norms are not optimal. Your blood levels are being compared to other men just as low as you are and if you fall within the bell curve, you are considered normal.

What is normal for you is not necessarily normal for another man. And that goes for women, too. We are not created equally. There is no perfect hormone level that fits all of us.

That's why you need to know your body. Or you can seek the professional assistance of a health care provider like me who knows hormones and their effect on your body, not just determine your hormonal health by your blood levels.

At the beach, it's easy to read the testosterone levels of the men around me. All they have to do is take off their shirts, turn around and let me look at the back of their arms. That muscle at the top of your arm is called the deltoid. The posterior deltoid at the back of the shoulder is testosterone driven. All young boys during their pubescent testosterone surge develop that muscle. It's very hard for women to develop the back of our deltoids. When male testosterone drops, the back of their arm flattens.

There have been studies showing that young fertile women are attracted to men with "strong" arms and shoulders. Why? Because they innately know that those men have enough testosterone to be fertile and to protect them. Now of course, we're talking about ancient biology that knows nothing of our technological world where you can buy infertility treatments and body guards.

Men's testosterone levels follow their mate's. If she is hormonally challenged, then he will soon follow her. I cannot tell you how many of my female patients bring their husbands in after their hormones are in balance. They got used to their mutually low sex drive, lack of motivation, poor sleep and general malaise. Once she feels better, she notices that he needs a tune-up.

Once your testosterone is back, whether it's through bioidentical hormone replacement therapy or natural support of testosterone production with Genesis Gold®, your life will change. You don't just get back your sex drive. You don't just lower your cholesterol levels. (Remember, steroid hormones are made by cholesterol, so normal testosterone for you means healthy cholesterol). You get your courage back.

Testosterone is the motivator. When your testosterone is low, you feel weaker, less able, more worried. When it is high, you feel strong, capable, motivated. This isn't just about sexual performance or muscle mass. For men, testosterone drives your sense of self.

One of my male patients told me he didn't realize how afraid he had become until after we balanced his hormones. He worked in downtown Los Angeles, in a rough part of the city. Once his testosterone levels were back up, he no longer rushed to the safety of his office. He held his head up, walking confidently to and from work, even after dark. Like the Cowardly Lion, he got his courage back.

NOW FOR THE SEX TALK

We think of testosterone as the sex hormone for both men and women. Yes, testosterone influences libido or sex drive. In men, testosterone also influences erectile function. In women, it's estrogen that influences sexual response.

Ladies, first of all, you need an understanding of your sexuality. Libido is your desire. Originating in your hypothalamus, libido is testosterone dependent. Arousal, your physical response, is estrogen dependent. Orgasm is a combination of all three hormones – estrogen, testosterone and progesterone.

From your responses to the following questions, your hormonal needs can be determined.

- Do you lubricate adequately for intercourse?

- Can you reach orgasm with your partner?

- Are you orgasmic by yourself?

- Is orgasm taking too long?

- Are you turned on by erotic reading or videos?

- How does your man smell to you?

Ladies, if your partner is no longer appealing and especially if he stinks when there has been no change in his personal hygiene habits, then I suspect your estrogen levels have dropped. Why?

Estrogen influences the sense of smell. It's why women are more attracted to perfumes and aromatic flowers. It's how women choose their best mates.

A study was done on college women. Half of them were taking birth control pills, the other half were not. They were given a bunch of T-shirts that had been worn by young men. The women were asked to choose the T-shirt they found most appealing by its odor. The fertile young women picked the T-shirts of the men that would be their best genetic match, meaning most likely to have healthy babies with those men. The women on birth control pills did not choose well. When you mess with natural hormone production, you interfere with your body's ability to guide you.

Now, men, that does not mean that personal hygiene is not important in attracting a mate. What it means is that women use their senses to choose their sex partners.

Men, it's your turn. I know you just want a magic pill that'll make you the man you used to be. Well, in spite of the commercials, erectile dysfunction drugs are not the answer. Let me ask you a couple of questions.

- Do you still wake up every morning with an erection?

  I know that seems a little personal, but if you don't, your testosterone levels are falling. Even if you do most mornings yet it's not like it was when you were a young man, then your testosterone is too low for you.

  All men have a spike of testosterone about an hour before dawn. Ask any man who works the graveyard shift. It doesn't matter if you're asleep or awake, when your testosterone spikes, your penis responds by filling with blood. You may have to urinate, but that need is not why you wake up with an erection.

- Do you have a family history of heart disease?

  If so, you best stay away from ED drugs, because if the blood isn't flowing to your penis adequately, your heart isn't getting all the blood it needs either. Arteriosclerosis needs to be ruled out before pumping you up with Viagra so you don't have a heart attack while making love.

What about sexual chemistry?

Through a kiss – not a peck, but a long deep kiss – you can tell a lot about a person. That is, if you're hormonally competent. Kissing is the best way to choose your genetic match. You're not just swapping spit, you're swapping DNA. If you're fertile, you experience sexual chemistry if there is a genetic match. You may be attracted to their physique, their eyes, their manners, their bank account. But if you don't think they're a good kisser, then don't make babies with them.

I had a patient's husband thank me for balancing his wife's hormones. He truly appreciated getting his wife back. She was happier, sleeping better and her sex drive had returned. He said, "I didn't realize how much had changed. I can tell her hormones are better. Now the skin of her arm responds to my lightest touch."

SO WHAT'S THE PAUSE?

Menopause is when a woman stops having periods.

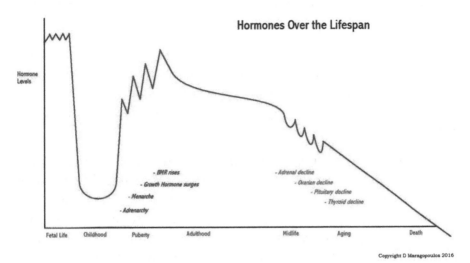

Hormones Over the Lifespan

Hormone Levels

- BMR rises
- Growth Hormone surges
- Menarche
- Adrenarchy

- Adrenal decline
- Ovarian decline
- Pituitary decline
- Thyroid decline

Fetal Life   Childhood   Puberty   Adulthood   Midlife   Aging   Death

Copyright D Maragopoulos 2016

Andropause is when a man's testosterone levels drop.

The average age of menopause is 51. Andropause is later. But the five to ten years prior to the pause, your hormones are declining. Not just your sex hormones – all your hormones. Women usually notice the changes. Men are just beginning to realize that their health issues may be related to their hormones.

As early as the mid 30's you experience a significant decline in adrenal function. Remember the adrenals need progesterone to make the stress hormone cortisol. So the stress of living our fast paced lives affects our hormones drastically. And yes, men make progesterone too, just not as much as women.

By age 40, most women have an 80% decline in progesterone levels. As progesterone declines, estrogen becomes dominant, leading to PMS, heavier periods, uterine fibroids, fibrocystic breasts, anxiety and depression. In their fourth decade, most men have a 25% decrease in their testosterone levels.

By age 50, most women have a 50% decline in estrogen levels. Low estrogen leads to loss of bone, hair, and nails, dry skin, mouth, eyes and vagina, less collagen formation leading to wrinkles, memory loss, hot flashes, night sweats, loss of bladder control, constipation and insomnia.

When estrogen first drops, more testosterone is left unbound which increases androgenic effects like acne and unwanted hair growth. But after menopause, most women experience a significant decrease in testosterone levels leading to bone and muscle loss, lack of motivation and low libido.

In their fifth decade, most men experience a 50% drop in their testosterone levels. Muscle is harder to build. Your waistline thickens. Your cholesterol levels rise. Your blood pressure may follow. You become anxious, less sure of yourself. You have trouble sleeping. You have less energy. You have to work way harder than ever to keep up with the younger guys in the gym, at work, in the bedroom.

You want your mojo back. And you want it now! But first we need to start with your gut.

CHAPTER 6

INSIDE OUT

Perimenopausal, tired and overweight, Cindy drove 300 miles to come and see me. She complained of the usual perimenopausal symptoms of fatigue, irritability, hot flashes, weight gain and no sex drive. Twice in the past few months, Cindy had been hospitalized with abdominal pain. Many tests later, the doctors could find nothing and sent Cindy home on pain meds. All she could eat was starches because everything else caused more pain. Now she was having trouble working as a bookkeeper because her joints ached constantly.

Cindy took my hand, "My sister-in-law said you could help me with my hormones."

I nodded, "I can, but you have a dysfunctional gut. Your stomach is not producing enough acid to break down protein, and the carbohydrate rich diet you've had to exist on is inflaming your joints. Until I fix your digestion, absorption and detoxification, I can't help you balance your hormones."

Of course, I could have given Cindy hormones to treat her perimenopausal symptoms, but that would have been a Band-Aid. My goal is to help you make your own hormones. And the primary way I do that is to feed your body what it needs to balance itself. If your gut is dysfunctional, you will not be able to absorb the micronutrients necessary to support your hypothalamus and keep your Hormones in Harmony®.

So we start with your gut.

YOU'RE A DONUT

Just like your skin protects you from the outer environment, the lining of your gut protects you from the inside. Like a donut, your outside reflects your inside. Unlike the skin, your gut has to let nutrients in and keep toxins out. It's a tall order. One you would think would be simple. Aren't you born with a healthy gut?

Well, if your mother had a perfectly healthy digestive tract colonized by a wide variety of beneficial bacteria, and she breastfed you for at least a year to prepare your infant intestines for the world, then yes, you probably started with a healthy gut.

But unless you've never taken antibiotics, whether prescribed or in your diet, and you've never taken antacids or aspirin or ibuprofen or any other nonsteroidal anti-inflammatory, and you eat naturally fermented foods every day, then perhaps you still have that pristine gut you were born with.

If not, we'd better focus on your gut.

Intestinal health is crucial to the proper functioning of your entire body.

That's why we begin with The **IN** cornerstone. It's how we fix everything else.

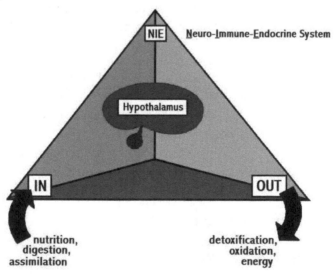

Biochemistry of the DMAR® Pyramid of Health

Under the Orchestration of the Hypothalamus, Hormones of the NIE sings to the DNA and the DNA dances

Copyright D Maragopoulos 2016

We are what we eat…literally.

We all know that protein builds muscle and that carbohydrates are energy foods. But did you know that every chemical you make – every hormone, every neurotransmitter, every cytokine – all come from nutrients derived from the food you eat?

If your diet does not provide all the nutrients necessary to run your system, then something has to go. Usually it's those parts of your body that are not crucial for life – your skin, your hair, your nails. Your internal health is directly related to your external appearance.

Hormones are made up of protein and fat…specifically cholesterol. In fact, "steroid" hormones are derived from the "sterol" in cholesterol. When you reach middle age and your hormones begin to decline, your cholesterol naturally rises in response. Your liver is just trying to help out your failing gonads!

Food is digested into protein, fat, and carbohydrates. These macronutrients provide calories and building blocks for new tissues and biochemicals like hormones. Micronutrients are the vitamins and minerals that help run the system. If you cannot digest your food properly, break it down into absorbable macronutrients and assimilate it into essential micronutrients, then you cannot produce adequate hormones to remain healthy.

Your liver and kidneys are organs that detoxify your body. They need energy from food (mostly carbohydrates) and essential amino acids (from protein) and essential fatty acids (from fats) to do their job. They also require micronutrients to run the detoxification pathways. It's an incredibly complicated system – one that most health care providers ignore.

Years ago, I was attending a medical conference. The physician presenter was lecturing on the drug interactions between a blood thinner and acetaminophen. After the lecture, I asked where in the hepatic detoxification pathways were the interactions occurring? When he didn't answer, I clarified by asking specifically about phase I enzyme interactions versus phase II conjugation issues.

As if I was speaking a different language, he said very slowly and very loudly, "I am a lung doctor, not a liver doctor."

I replied, "Doctor, don't all your 'lung' patients have livers? So wouldn't it behoove you and your patients to know what detoxification pathways are affected? That way you can advise your patients on what foods, herbs, and supplements to also avoid."

He shook his head. "I just check their blood levels frequently."

And his patients are dependent on him not to bleed to death!

Now, I know that as a layperson, you probably do not have a clue about the hepatic detoxification pathways, but I expected my esteemed colleague to understand. We learned this basic physiology in our undergraduate pre-med training. Yet so few of us utilize knowledge of biochemistry in our clinical practices. And it is **SO VERY IMPORTANT!**

That's why, as a patient, you need to know how your body works so you can make the healthiest choices. Knowledge is power and very well may save your life.

LET'S TAKE A TOUR OF YOUR GUT

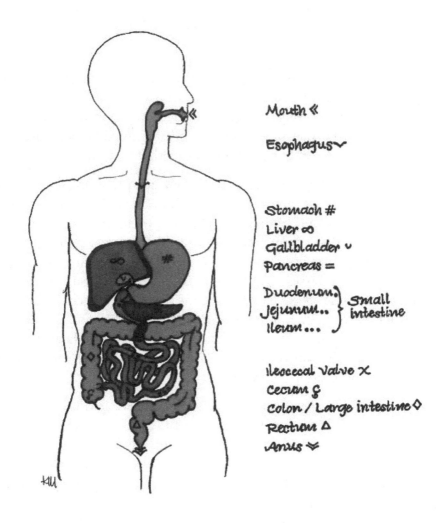

Mouth «

Esophagus ⌄

Stomach #
Liver ∞
Gallbladder ⌄
Pancreas =

Duodenum 🙂
Jejunum.. } Small intestine
Ileum ...

Ileocecal valve ✗
Cecum §
Colon / Large intestine ◇
Rectum △
Anus ⌄⌄

Let's say you eat a peanut butter and jelly sandwich. I know it's not exactly health food, but bear with me. Just looking at that delicious PB&J, you begin salivating. Your salivary glands are exocrine glands. Unlike endocrine glands that produce hormones that are carried by the bloodstream to cells all over your body, exocrine glands act locally.

As soon as you take that first bite of your delicious PB&J, the enzyme in your saliva called amylase breaks down the sugars in the jelly and the starches in bread. Right through your mouth, you absorb the sugar. You don't even have to swallow to get your first hit of calories!

That sugar goes directly into your bloodstream and right to your hypothalamus. Remember, your brain loves sugar and your hypothalamus is no exception. Your hypothalamus produces dopamine in response to that lovely sugar. Dopamine is the neurotransmitter that fuels the reward center of your brain. Your hypothalamus ensures that you don't forget to eat by rewarding you with dopamine.

A dopamine surge also happens in your gut, preparing it for action. Your stomach begins ramping up hydrochloride acid production to get ready for that peanut butter and jelly sandwich. Your first few bites slide down your esophagus, let's say, with the help of a tall glass of milk. Your esophagus is a long tube that connects your mouth and throat to your stomach. It passes right by your heart, through your diaphragm, ending in a peptic sphincter which opens into the stomach. Your peptic sphincter keeps your food and your gastric acid in your stomach. If gastric acid leaks up into the esophagus, you experience heartburn. It's not your heart that's burning. It's your esophagus that is being burnt by the highly acidic stomach acid.

Gastric acid is very, very acidic. Hydrochloric acid is a pH of 1.0. In comparison, water is neutral at a pH of 7.0. Your stomach protects itself from this highly acidic acid by producing mucus. It's like a sea anemone. Have you ever touched a sea anemone? This little flower shaped sea creature that lives in tide pools has a sticky mucusy surface that protects it from the acid it uses to digest the little fishes that get caught in its mouth tendrils. Your stomach makes that same type of mucus. Gastritis happens not when you make too much stomach acid, but when your mucin cells are damaged and your stomach cannot make enough mucus to protect itself.

If you take antacids to neutralize your stomach acid or H2 blockers to reduce stomach acid production, you temporarily protect your stomach from the burn, but you will not be able to digest protein. You will be like Cindy – only able to digest pure sugar and starches.

And if you don't burn all the energy from that pure sugar, you will store it in your body fat. That's how Cindy became obese. Because she had abdominal pain, her doctors gave her H2 blockers like Pepcid or Prilosec, and guess what, she couldn't digest protein.

Cindy had stomach pain to start with, not because she made too much acid, but because she made too little gastric acid. She was hypochloric. I treated Cindy by healing the mucin cells of her stomach to make enough acid to digest protein and enough mucus to protect herself from her own gastric acid. Then she could stop eating sugar and starches and start eating protein and vegetables. And guess what? She lost weight!

You need lots of gastric acid to digest your food properly. Unless you're eating pure sugar or processed starches like white flour, all your food has a protein matrix which must be broken down by stomach acid. Once the acid breaks down the protein, that PB&J, now called chyme, is dumped through the pyloric sphincter into the first part of your small intestine called the duodenum.

Since the chyme is highly acidic at a pH of 1.0, your duodenum needs to be protected. Here comes bile to your rescue! Your liver produces bile, which is very alkaline at a pH of 9.0. Bile is stored in your gallbladder. As soon as the chyme arrives in your small intestine, the broken down protein and fat causes a gut hormone called cholecystokinin to be released. Cholecystokinin tells your gallbladder to dump the bile.

Your gallbladder duct opens into the duodenum right under the pyloric sphincter. The very alkaline bile neutralizes the very acidic chyme. Now your partially digested food is at a neutral pH of 6.8-7.2, which is exactly what it needs to be at for your digestive enzymes to work.

Your pancreas is responsible for producing digestive enzymes. I know I told you that your pancreas is an endocrine gland that produces hormones, but it also is an exocrine gland that produces enzymes. And those enzymes are dumped directly into the duodenum. Your pancreas produces eight cups of enzyme-rich pancreatic juice every day to help you digest your foods.

Pancreatic enzymes do not work alone. They need beneficial bacteria. Your small intestine harbors billions of beneficial bacteria, specifically Bifidus. These bacteria help you digest your food and activate the vitamins in your food so you can use them. That's why they're called beneficial bacteria. Without these billions of little guys, you could not survive.

Now your small intestine is really, really long – about 24 feet in length. It takes that much surface area to absorb the nutrients from your food. Most of digestion occurs in the duodenum at the beginning of the small intestinal tract. Absorption occurs in the middle, called the jejunum. This part of your small intestine is connected to a rich network of blood called the mesentery. The macronutrients from your PB&J – amino acids, fatty acids and sugars – along with the micronutrients – vitamins and minerals – are absorbed through your jejunum into the mesentery arteries and go to the liver. What also gets absorbed are any toxins in your food – like herbicides sprayed on the wheat.

Your liver then has to filter the good from the bad. It processes the nutrients and sends them into the bloodstream for the cells of your body to use. Your liver also breaks down the toxins and handcuffs them to be dumped back into the bile and released out through the colon. This is the part that the lung doctor I mentioned earlier forgot. Bogging down your liver with lots of drugs makes it have to work that much harder.

Your liver also filters hormones from your bloodstream that are done doing their job. Those hormones are also handcuffed in a process called conjugation. If your small intestine has healthy beneficial bacteria, then your handcuffed hormones are defecated out. If you don't have enough beneficial bacteria, the other microbes in your intestine take over like gangsters.

These gangster microbes produce enzymes that take the handcuffs right off the hormones and toxins and they're reabsorbed back into the bloodstream. Your intestine no longer does a good job of absorbing nutrients.

Now what's left over from your PB&J is passed on to the end of your small intestine called the ileum through the ileocecal valve and into your colon.

Your colon is called the large intestine because it is much bigger in diameter than the small intestine. Your colon is rich with its own flora – friendly bacteria, mostly Lactobacillus and E. coli.

Now there's many, many more bacteria species in your gut. The more diverse your gut flora is, the healthier you are. Variety is the spice of life. And you need lots of diversity in your gut microbes to stay healthy and keep your immune system functioning well.

Your colon's job is to compact your undigested food and get it out as feces. Your colon can pull water from your blood stream to make hard fecal matter soft and it can push water out to make loose feces firm. Your colon has a very intelligent transpermeable membrane. It only allows tiny water molecules in and out. If your colon is damaged, it becomes leaky, allowing toxins and undigested food particles to escape into the bloodstream. These bypass the liver and become irritants. Your body responds to your leaky gut by making lots of antibodies. You develop food allergies. You begin attacking yourself. This is called autoimmunity.

Your PB&J's journey ends in the rectum where it is defecated out as stool. It takes about eight hours for what you put into your mouth to pass through your entire digestive tract and out through your anus. If it takes much longer, you experience constipation. If it is rapid, you experience diarrhea.

I once had a couple who both suffered with Irritable Bowel Syndrome. One had severe abdominal pain and frequent diarrhea. One had cramping, bloating and constipation. I recommended Genesis Gold® for both of them. They each got better. How can one thing fix both problems?

Because your gastrointestinal tract functions with a rich network of neuro-endocrine hormones. I only mentioned a few, but there are many, many more hormones that control your digestion and absorption.

Genesis Gold® balances the entire neuro-immune-endocrine system, including the hormones that control your gut health. Conventional medicine often prescribes anti-anxiety or anti-depressants for Irritable Bowel Syndrome. The drugs are Band-Aids, not cures. Getting to the root of the issue by healing the miscommunication within your neuro-immune-endocrine system is how Genesis Gold® works.

WHEN YOUR GUT MAKES YOU ANXIOUS

Remember, your gut is your second brain. And it influences the brain in your head.

Mitch came to me with severe anxiety. He had been suffering from panic attacks, insomnia and generalized anxiety for months. His doctors had given him anti-anxiety meds but he wanted off. He wanted his life back.

As a professional artist, Mitch found the treatment to be nearly as debilitating as the panic attacks. Like the Scarecrow, Mitch felt like his brain wasn't working. The drugs blocked his creative abilities so much so that he couldn't work, he couldn't support himself, and that made him more depressed, more anxious.

This wasn't the first time Mitch had had debilitating panic attacks. I asked him if he had ever been treated with antibiotics. As a matter of fact, he had – both times he had panic attacks. Mitch had been treated for prostatitis with a long heavy course of antibiotics twice. And twice he had severe panic attacks that sent him into the emergency room.

The antibiotics killed off all of Mitch's gut bacteria. Without his beneficial bacteria, Mitch's gut began producing some anxiety-inducing hormones. His hypothalamus got wind of the havoc in his gut and triggered Mitch's brain to go into survival mode. Without a real enemy to fight or flee, Mitch experienced severe anxiety and panic attacks.

So we healed his gut with a regimen designed to eradicate the gangster microbes, repair his leaky gut lining, and replenish his beneficial gut flora. Plus, we healed his hypothalamic imbalance with Genesis Gold® and got him off the drugs.

Mitch called a couple months later to thank me. His blood tests had improved so much, his doctor said to continue whatever he was doing. No more drugs – just healthy diet, lifestyle, and Genesis Gold®.

CHAPTER 7

STRESS AND THE SWEET THIEF

Sally came to me complaining of hair loss. She had tried everything – every hair growth product on the market, every prescription to treat hair loss, every supplement to help grow hair. At 38, she only had half her hair left.

Sally had been losing hair for the past ten years. I asked her what happened ten years ago. She described a major life change which included a career shift while involved in an abusive relationship. She also described a very stressful childhood. Poor lifestyle choices during the formative years of her adolescence led to malnutrition, toxicity, and living in a constant state of fear.

By her mid-twenties, Sally had gotten her life together. She was living well, making good money, described some supportive friends. Yet she was programmed from childhood to respond to life in perpetual fight or flight mode. And her body, specifically her hair, was paying the price.

STRESS MAKES YOU SICK

Stress – a fact of modern day living and the cause of so many diseases. Stress has been linked to heart disease, cancer, allergies, autoimmune disease, thyroid dysfunction, mood disorders and obesity.

While stress affects many parts of the body, the adrenals are responsible for creating the stress response. The adrenals are small glands that lie on top of your kidneys. These amazing glands have multiple functions.

The adrenal glands control blood pressure, orchestrate protein, fat, and carbohydrate metabolism, influence the immune system and run the stress response.

That's a lot of responsibility for one pair of glands.

Take a look at all your adrenal glands do:

Adrenal Gland

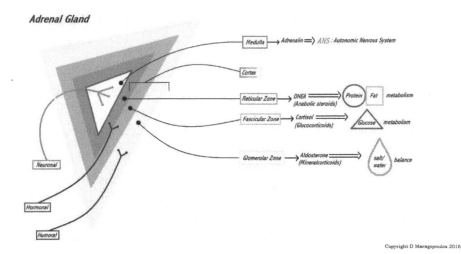

So what happens when you're under stress?

First, your adrenals are stimulated by the nervous system (neuronal) and the adrenal medulla produces adrenaline. Adrenaline increases your heart rate and blood pressure to initiate the fight or flight response.

Then your adrenals are stimulated by the hypothalamic-pituitary-axis (hormonal) and the adrenal cortex produces cortisol to fuel the fight or flight response.

Your adrenals respond to the electrolytes in your blood (humoral) and the outer part of the adrenal cortex produces aldosterone that controls your blood pressure by balancing salt/water output by the kidneys.

Cortisol is a catabolic steroid hormone. Catabolic = breaks down. Steroid = made from cholesterol. Hormone = chemical messenger.

Cortisol fuels the stress response and then it breaks down other tissues – skin, hair, nails, muscles, and organs. Bones break down, leading to osteoporosis. Even the gut lining is affected by high levels of cortisol leading to leaky gut syndrome, food allergies and malabsorption.

Like most endocrine glands, your adrenals are stimulated by the hypothalamic-pituitary axis in a negative feedback system. Think of a seesaw. Cortisol is on one side and adrenal-cortico-trophic hormone (ACTH) is on the other. If cortisol is high, ACTH is low. If cortisol is low, ACTH is high.

The Stress Response

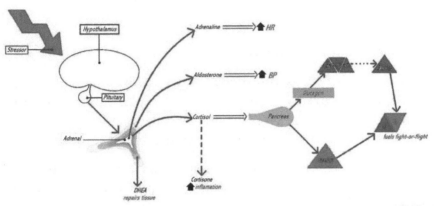

Let's say a tiger is chasing you. Your autonomic nervous system stimulates the adrenals to produce adrenaline. Your heart beats faster raising your blood pressure so you can get away. The adrenaline surge stimulates your hypothalamus which checks to see if you have enough cortisol to fuel the stress response. If not, your hypothalamus tells the pituitary gland to produce ACTH, which travels via the blood stream to the adrenal cortex and stimulates the production of cortisol.

Cortisol then tells the pancreas to produce glucagon, which is the hormone that releases glycogen (stored sugar) from the muscles and the liver. Now your muscles and heart have the energy to get away from that tiger!

Whew! Following the surge of cortisol, the adrenals produce dehydroepiandrosterone, also known as DHEA. DHEA controls protein and fat metabolism to help repair the damage from the flight or fight. The leftover cortisol is converted to cortisone, a natural anti-inflammatory, to soothe your aches after getting away from the tiger.

At first the high stress response causes a catabolic reaction as your tissues break down. You might lose weight initially, but over the long haul, the high levels of cortisol can cause you to store body fat. Remember, cortisol stimulates the release of stored sugar. How can the glucose get into the cells without insulin? So the pancreas also produces more insulin in response to the stress. If you are really running away from the tiger, then of course, you will use the glucose.

If not, if you're lucky, you develop insulin resistance.

What's Insulin Resistance?

Insulin resistance is your body's way of protecting itself from all that circulating sugar. Too much sugar is very inflammatory. Insulin resistance is major cause of cardiovascular inflammation and hardening of the arteries, leading to stroke, heart attacks and death.

Insulin escorts glucose into the cells. Cells use glucose to produce energy. If the tiger is not really chasing you and you are not expending the energy, then your cells become resistant to insulin. All cells that cannot store sugar become insulin resistant. Your liver and muscles can store about 400 calories worth of glucose. Your heart, on the other hand, cannot store even one gram of sugar.

Make a fist. That's the size of an efficient heart for your body. Your heart can only use glucose to beat faster or grow bigger. A bigger heart is not an efficient pump, so your heart becomes insulin resistant.

What does your body do with the extra sugar? It stores it as fat. Thankfully, your adipose (fat) cells never become insulin resistant. No, they will store that extra sugar in the form of triglycerides (triple sugar molecules) to protect the rest of your body.

Insulin resistance is why you end up gaining weight after prolonged stress.

INSULIN RESISTANCE – THE PATH TO OBESITY AND DIABETES

There are two types of diabetes: Type 1 and Type 2. Type 1 Diabetes, also known as juvenile diabetes, is an autoimmune disease that damages the pancreas so it cannot produce insulin. Type 1 Diabetics are insulin dependent. They must take insulin to survive. Type 2 Diabetes occurs when your cells no longer allow insulin in. Your pancreas makes more than enough insulin, in fact too much, but insulin doesn't work properly. We call this Insulin Resistance.

Insulin is a hormone produced by the pancreas that escorts glucose (sugar) into your cells for energy production. Hormones need receptor sites in the cell membrane to work. Every cell on your body has insulin receptors.

My daughter created this graphic for me to teach you about hormones. Kyra was taking pre-nursing courses at the time and said that after creating my Hormone in Harmony® graphics, she could understand cell biology much better.

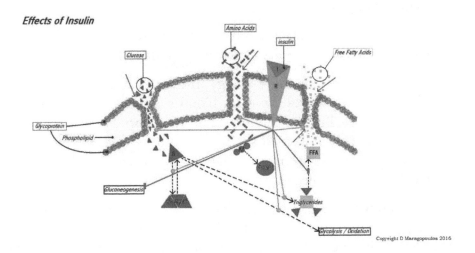

Effects of Insulin

Copyright D Maragopoulos 2016

You can see in the above graphic that the cell membrane is made up of glycoprotein and phospholipids with receptor sites that allow hormones to interact with the cell. Glycoproteins are sugars bonded to protein that make up the inner and outer cell membrane. Phospholipids are fats that act as an insulating layer between the glycoprotein layers and provide space for cell receptor sites.

Receptor sites are very specific. Estrogen receptor sites only allow estrogen into the cell. Cortisol receptor sites only allow cortisol into the cell. Unlike steroid receptor sites, insulin receptors act like a lock and key. The insulin receptor is the lock and insulin is the key.

Insulin escorts glucose to your cells. When insulin docks onto the cell receptor, it opens a gateway for glucose to get into the cell. But it does so much more. Insulin also opens an amino acid gateway so the cell has protein building blocks to make more of what it needs, a free fatty acid gateway to help the cell make fats like triglycerides or fats to repair the cell membrane and create healthy receptor sites for hormones, and a water gate that hydrates the cell.

When the insulin receptors are functioning, your cells do not have to break down their own fats and protein for energy (gluconeogenesis). Instead your cells package the incoming glucose into glycogen. Then when the cell needs energy, it breaks down the stored glycogen back into glucose (glycolysis).

If you're insulin resistant, you're not just missing glucose, you're malnourished. Your cells are not getting protein, fats, or water!

When you consume more energy in calories than you expend in activity, your body stores the extra blood sugar as glycogen in your liver and muscles. But you can only store 400 calories of glycogen (the amount of calories in a small sandwich). The rest of the extra sugar is repackaged by the liver into triglycerides which are three sugar molecules on a fat molecule.

Your body then stores all the triglycerides in the only cells that can receive the extra sugar – your fat cells. The fat cells most receptive to storage are the ones around your middle. The fat around your middle is called your "insulin meter".

Do you have an Insulin Meter?

The thicker your waist is in comparison to your hips, the more likely you are insulin resistant. That's why waist circumference is a much better way to measure your fat storage than BMI (body mass index). Unfortunately, BMI is used by insurance companies to determine obesity. Very lean professional football players have extremely high BMIs and would be considered obese, and of course they aren't.

Even the clothing industry has changed its proportions to match America's expanding waistlines. Years ago, I was costuming my daughter's drama class for its winter production. I had a high-waist red business suit that looked like it should fit the fifteen-year-old who was playing the mother. While this girl was quite thin, I had to expand the waist in the pants to fit her. She was not an exception.

Since the mid-nineties, our youth's waistlines have been expanding – corresponding to our computer technology when kids began to spend much less time playing outdoors and more time in front of screens.

Most doctors do not treat Insulin Resistance. Treatment usually starts when a patient is diagnosed as Diabetic. Why wait?

Are you at risk for Insulin Resistance?

Before you become frankly diabetic, there's a marker in your blood that starts to rise called c-peptide. I measure c-peptide in my patients to determine their risk for insulin resistance.

C-peptide is a protein molecule that is produced by the pancreas and binds insulin to pro-insulin. While the pancreas produces enzymes to help you digest your food, it is also an endocrine gland that produces hormones – insulin and glucagon – that are transported by the blood to all the cells of your body. Insulin gets sugar into the cells. Glucagon gets sugar out.

Once released in the bloodstream, the triple complex of insulin~c-peptide~pro-insulin splits. The pancreas reuptakes pro-insulin to make more insulin. Insulin binds with blood glucose to escort it into the cells for energy production. C-peptide floats freely in the blood.

C-peptide reflects how much insulin your pancreas is producing. Type 1 Diabetics produce no insulin so their c-peptide is not measurable. As you become more insulin resistant, your pancreas produces more insulin. C-peptide levels rise. The higher your c-peptide, the more insulin you are producing. Over years of producing too much insulin, the pancreas becomes exhausted and eventually patients with Type 2 Diabetes may need to take insulin.

You are Who You Live With

For over twenty years, I have been counseling couples and families on lifestyle changes to treat Diabetes and Insulin Resistance. These "diseases" are more nurture than nature – more about your lifestyle choices than your family history.

Yes, you may have a tendency to develop diabetes at middle age because your mother or father has it, but that's just a tendency. You were not born with Type 2 Diabetes. You develop it over time, after years of poor lifestyle choices...that you, your partner, and your entire family share.

Remember, DNA is like a deck of playing cards. You are dealt a lot of cards, some good, some bad, but it's how you play those cards that determines the outcome of the game. Same with DNA. You're born with lots of DNA, most of which is not expressed.

It's how you play the game of life and the choices you make. What you eat, how active you are, do you get enough sleep, and your attitude (yes, if you assume the worst, you manifest it and vice versa) – all these choices overtime determine the outcome of your health. It's best to start early, but it's never too late! You can change anything...even your health...even reverse Type 2 Diabetes.

I find that most of my middle-aged couples have nearly identical blood markers for insulin resistance. They're not related, but they are living the same life.

A recent study found that the partners of type II diabetics have a 26% increased risk of developing diabetes. These partners studied shared the same poor diets, sleep habits, lack of physical activity, stressors and exposure to nocturnal light.

Since your family shares eating and activity habits as well as belief systems, I believe treating the whole family is the only way to treat the growing problem of Insulin Resistance.

WHAT IF THE STRESS NEVER ENDS?

Remember, I said, if you're lucky, you get insulin resistant? It's how your hypothalamus saves you from your stressful life. That weight gain around your middle is like a buoy helping you float through the stressors of your life. Your hypothalamus is just helping you survive until the world is safe. If you get treed by that tiger, then you can survive on that extra fat you've stored around your middle!

Now in the wild, you would either get eaten by the tiger or out smart it. You would not be chased forever. Today stressors are constant.

The hypothalamus does not know the difference between a tiger chasing you and you being late for work. The adrenal response is the same: Adrenaline —> Cortisol —> DHEA. Over and over and over again, day after day, week after week, for months, maybe years on end, the stress of modern day life puts a toll on the adrenals. Eventually they become fatigued, producing less and less cortisol and DHEA until you can hardly function.

What are the symptoms of Adrenal Fatigue?

- **Profound fatigue** - You struggle to wake up in the morning. You need caffeine and sugar to start your day. Your energy crashes in the afternoon. Sometimes you get a second wind at night and cannot sleep. This is a reversed circadian rhythm and it's usually early in the course of adrenal dysfunction.

- **Unhealthy Skin, Hair and Nails** - The early stress response creates high DHEA production which converts to testosterone and then dihydrotestosterone causing hair loss. Then your adrenals get so exhausted, your DHEA production bottoms out. Your hair is thin, dry, brittle. Your nails are brittle and slow growing. Your skin is dry and aging fast, although early in the stress response the high cortisol levels will induce oily, acne prone skin. Wounds heal very slowly. This is partially because of the catabolic nature of cortisol and mostly because of the decreased production of DHEA that normally helps you metabolize protein and fat to grow new you (hair, skin, nails and other more important tissues). If your hair, skin and nails are unhealthy, you can bet that your internal organs do not look so good.

- **You're sick a lot** - You cannot seem to recover from illnesses. You keep catching one cold after another. All your old viruses come back to haunt you. You break out in cold sores, genital warts, relapse with chronic infections like Epstein Barr and hepatitis. Your immune system does not seem to be working properly.

- **Sugar Cravings** - When you eat, cortisol is produced which releases stored sugar so that you have immediate fuel until your food is digested. Tired adrenal glands do not produce enough cortisol and you crave sugar after you eat.

- **Salt Cravings** - Your adrenals also make another hormone called aldosterone that regulates salt water balance. Fatigued adrenals do not produce enough aldosterone, so your blood pressure is low. You get up too fast and you feel dizzy. Healthy adrenals produce enough aldosterone to raise your blood pressure twenty points when you rise from a lying to a standing position. Otherwise if you were napping under a tree, how would you be able to get away from that tiger?

- **Slow Metabolism** - Eventually your thyroid is affected. That's because thyroid function is controlled by the same hypothalamic hormone (POMC) as the adrenal glands.

- **Sex Hormones Decline** - That's because reproduction is not a necessary function when your body is under profound stress. Most brides experience this stress response when their period shows up on their wedding day. Your adrenals use progesterone to make cortisol. Progesterone stabilizes the lining of the uterus. High stress equals high cortisol production and there is not enough progesterone to regulate the menstrual cycle. Eventually, inadequately opposed estrogen leads to heavy, painful periods and fibroids. Overtime, your imbalanced sex hormones induce early menopausal and andropausal symptoms. Yes, stress affects men, too.

Conventional medicine does not recognize adrenal fatigue. Why? Because while adrenal fatigue is not optimal functioning, it is not a disease. Complete adrenal failure is called Addison's disease. Your adrenal glands no longer produce cortisol. You need cortisol to survive, so you are given synthetic cortisone for the rest of your life.

Why wait until you have full blown Addison's disease? Why not stop before you fall off the cliff?

Integrative medicine recognizes less than optimal functioning as something that can be improved through better lifestyle choices, detoxification, and supplementation.

Adrenal fatigue is recognized by integrative medicine as a treatable condition.

Adaptogenic herbs, B vitamins, essential fatty acids can help adrenal glands recover. Glandular products are useful initially to support adrenal function, but you weren't meant to eat hormones and glandulars are rich in hormones. After six months or so, your liver treats glandular supplements as toxic. They no longer support the gland.

Sometimes bio-identical cortisol and DHEA can be prescribed to supplement adrenal function, but again only until the adrenals can function on their own. So natural breaks to wake up the hypothalamic-pituitary-adrenal axis are crucial if your adrenals are ever going to make their own hormones. Bio-identicals are great, but nothing matches natural hormonal production that follows the seasons and your unique stress response.

I believe the body will heal itself given the proper nutrients. So first I recommend foundational support to heal the adrenals as well as all the organ systems affected by stress. Getting the adrenals functioning properly will stop the hair loss, weight gain, and aging, but the body needs extra nutrients to grow hair and healthy skin, improve body composition to increase lean body mass and decrease body fat, and optimize health.

I always recommend hypothalamic support to improve the communication system between the adrenals and the brain. Supporting the hypothalamus allows it to orchestrate the rest of the endocrine system as well as the neurological and immune system to harmonize the symphony of hormones, neurotransmitters and cytokines so your DNA dances optimal health and wellbeing.

Yes, I recommend adrenal glandulars and adaptogenic herbs for a few months to boost adrenal activity, but revving the engine without providing gas and oil will burn out the vehicle.

Genesis Gold® is the fuel that provides foundational support for your adrenal glands as well as optimizes your hypothalamic-pituitary-adrenal axis.

Remember Sally?

To stop her hair loss and increase hair growth, I helped Sally reprogram her stress response with a holistic mind-body approach.

First, she got foundational and hypothalamic support with Genesis Gold®. Then I treated her hormone imbalance through lifestyle counseling. More nutritious foods, better sleep hygiene, consistent circadian activity. I prescribed some topical hormones to promote her hair growth until she could make the necessary adjustments to her life. And through all this, I counseled her regarding her programmed stress response. Over time, as she completed the homework, made the lifestyle changes, and reprogrammed her subconscious, Sally got healthy.

Most people describe a more Zen approach to life when taking Genesis Gold®. One middle-aged male patient described a new found ability to take a higher perspective when dealing with stressful family situations since he started Genesis Gold®.

Years ago, my husband was asked what Genesis Gold® did for him. He said he felt more mellow. We all noticed the change, even the dogs. When he would pay bills he would get so uptight that the dogs would hide. Now they lie happily at my husband's feet as he navigates the monthly bills!

Physically, his waistline slimmed and he looks younger – the benefits of a healthier metabolism and less stressed attitude. Of course, I was happy he was taking better care of himself, especially since he worked for 30 years as a police officer – such a high stress job that within a few years of retirement many cops suffer heart attacks and die. He's been consistent with taking Genesis Gold® since 2008 and it shows. Even in his mid-fifties, his lab tests are that of a healthy thirty-year-old.

CHAPTER 8

PROTECTING YOURSELF

Brenda came to me tired and wired. After three years of infertility treatments, she was thrilled to conceive twins. She was on bedrest in her last trimester and had help once she gave birth four weeks early, but she never recovered her pre-pregnancy energy levels. Although the toddlers were sleeping through the night, Brenda had trouble falling asleep and woke up frequently. She woke up anxious and had trouble eating because her stomach was upset. Once the twins were up, she was afraid to sit still because she frequently dozed off, so she just kept moving. Brenda was running on fumes.

Upon palpating Brenda's neck, I found her thyroid was enlarged. Shaped like a butterfly, the thyroid gland wraps its wing-like lobes behind the trachea at the base of the neck.

I love the thyroid! It's the perfect endocrine gland to illustrate the negative feedback system of hormones. Check out this cool graphic my daughter made:

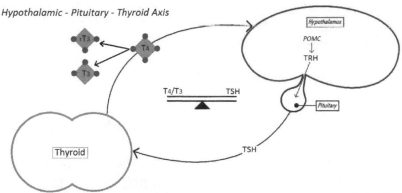

Hypothalamic - Pituitary - Thyroid Axis

Remember the hypothalamic hormone POMC? That's the great big hormone that controls your thyroid, your adrenals, your glucose metabolism, and your mood. We may be focusing on the thyroid right now, but I always check the rest of the hormones to be sure the other endocrine glands are healthy.

In the diagram, you can see your hypothalamus produces POMC in response to the circulating thyroid hormones – T4 and T3. POMC breaks down to TRH – Thyroid Releasing Hormone, which tells your pituitary gland to produce TSH – Thyroid Stimulating Hormone.

Notice the seesaw with TSH on one side and T4 and T3 on the other. If your thyroid hormone production is low, your TSH will be high. This is called hypothyroidism. And vice versa, if your thyroid hormone production is high, your TSH will be low. This is called hyperthyroidism.

Your thyroid's job is to make hormones that do one thing – control your metabolism.

Your thyroid makes thyroxine, known as T4 because it has four iodine molecules. T4 is not the hormone that controls your metabolism. T3 – triiodothyronine – is the active thyroid hormone.

Not all T3 molecules are equally effective. If the wrong iodine molecule is removed, it is called reverse T3 (rT3) and is not active. Oh, rT3 fits in the thyroid hormone receptor on your cells, but it doesn't open the lock. Reverse T3 is a dummy key. Only active T3 can open the lock, get into your cells, and tell your mitochondria to make more energy.

Typically only TSH, T4 and total T3 are measured when you get blood work, but that doesn't tell you the real picture. Only your unbound thyroid hormone is active. We call that unbound hormone free, as in free T4 (fT4) and free T3 (fT3). You need to know what your fT4, fT3, and rT3 levels are in comparison to your TSH.

But what if your TSH and your fT4 and fT3 are low? Or both high? That's miscommunication between your hypothalamus, your pituitary, and your thyroid. It's called your hypothalamic-pituitary-thyroid axis or HPT axis. And you can see this level of HPT miscommunication before your labs register too low or too high. You can be within normal limits, but have HPT axis miscommunication and you will have symptoms of thyroid problems. And you will be told that there's nothing wrong, that your labs are normal.

That's what happened to Brenda. She was told that there was nothing wrong, that her labs were fine. But she didn't feel fine, so she came to see me.

Brenda's thyroid levels were low when she became pregnant, but never treated. That always concerns me because babies born to a mother with low thyroid function often have developmental delays. The fetal brain needs healthy maternal hormones to develop properly.

I wish every young woman would receive pre-conceptual counseling. The healthier she is, the healthier her babies will be. As the Hormone Queen®, I've helped many infertile women conceive. My goal is to get them as healthy as possible – Their guts healthy, their immune system strong, their Hormones in Harmony® – before getting pregnant.

Within a few months of taking Genesis Gold®, most of my infertile patients conceive without infertility treatment, even those who needed artificial insemination or in vitro fertilization to conceive their first child. And their pregnancies on Genesis Gold® are healthier – no gestational diabetes, no hypertension, no excessive weight gain, easier deliveries.

One of my infertile patients conceived her first child with conventional medical assistance and her second child naturally with my help. Her first child has learning disabilities; her second child does not. She attributes it to Genesis Gold®. I attribute it to getting her optimally healthy before conceiving.

ATTACKING YOURSELF

I suspected Brenda suffered from thyroiditis. And her labs confirmed my suspicion. Her TSH and free T4/T3 levels were all low, meaning she had miscommunication in her HPT axis. Her thyroid had been functioning at such a low level for so long that her TSH was no longer responding. It's like her pituitary gland had given up. But more concerning were her high antibodies.

Brenda's body was making antibodies against her own thyroid hormone production. The attack on her own thyroid was causing it to swell with inflammation. Her enlarged thyroid often made swallowing difficult. She noticed her voice was a little hoarse. That's because her enlarged thyroid was pressing on her vocal cords.

Thyroiditis is an autoimmune condition. Autoimmunity means you are attacking yourself.

Thyroiditis is often called Hashimoto's thyroiditis after the physician who first discovered the condition. Conventional medicine treats thyroiditis with synthetic thyroid hormone, but that doesn't treat the cause.

Once started on thyroid hormone, patients often become dependent for life on thyroid replacement therapy. Why? Because if you're taking something your body should be making, that gland becomes lazy. It's like spraining your ankle and then wearing a brace for the rest of your life. You never strengthen the joint if you don't take off the support and exercise it.

I prefer to strengthen my patients' endocrine glands, to help them make their own hormones. That doesn't mean I won't offer them hormone replacement if they are low. I just give it in a way that teaches the failing gland to make its own hormones. And I always support their hypothalamus. Because without hypothalamic support, the hormonal miscommunication will continue.

Autoimmune antibodies are elevated in thyroiditis. TPO – thyroid peroxidase – antibodies are the most commonly elevated. These antibodies destroy the enzymes necessary to convert the large protein molecule called thyroglobulin into thyroid hormone.

Conventional treatment is designed to suppress TSH with enough synthetic thyroid hormone and hopefully suppress thyroid enzyme production to suppress antibody production. The result is lifelong dependency on thyroid hormone replacement therapy. The antibody levels take a very long time to normalize, if ever, using conventional therapy.

Thyroid Replacement Therapy (TRT) includes synthetic thyroxine (T4) and occasionally synthetic lieothyrodine (T3), as well as animal derived T4 and T3 (Armour Thyroid). Bio-identical botanically derived thyroid hormone (both T3 & T4) can be compounded by a qualified compounding pharmacist. Only bio-identical TRT can be delivered transdermally or sublingually. Synthetics and glandulars must be taken orally.

Focusing on the hypothalamic-pituitary-thyroid axis is crucial in lowering the damaging anti-thyroid antibodies. The specially formulated Sacred Seven® amino acids in Genesis Gold® optimizes hypothalamic communication and lowers antithyroid antibodies much more rapidly than with thyroid replacement therapy alone. In some cases of thyroiditis with normal thyroid hormone production and elevated antithyroid antibodies, I have found Genesis Gold® alone to be highly effective.

YOUR BODY TRIES TO PROTECT ITSELF

Your immune system's job is to protect you. Your bone marrow produces the soldiers – your white blood cells (WBC). These young WBCs must be trained, so they go to the thymus for boot camp. Then your trained WBCs travel around your body looking for invaders. They depend on your tonsils, appendix, and lymph nodes to hold onto any suspicious organisms. Once your WBCs capture the invaders, they travel to your spleen. In your spleen, your WBCs are debriefed. The information regarding the safety of your body is then communicated to the thymus via cytokines – the tiniest of hormones.

The Anatomy of the Immune System

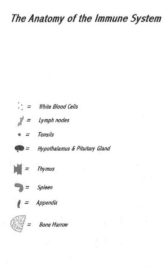

: = White Blood Cells

= Lymph nodes

• = Tonsils

= Hypothalamus & Pituitary Gland

= Thymus

= Spleen

= Appendix

= Bone Marrow

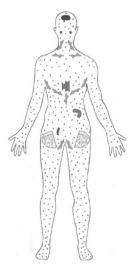

Copyright D Maragopoulos 2016

The white blood cells are specifically programmed by your thymus to know the difference between you and other.

Your hypothalamus controls your immune system. At night your hypothalamus triggers your pituitary gland to produce a hormone called prolactin. Prolactin triggers your thymus to program white blood cells known as lymphocytes to know the difference between you and other.

Other is any bacteria, fungi, virus, or mutant cancer cell. Your trained lymphocytes, called T-cells, know how to tell the difference between your normal healthy body cells and foreign cells.

In autoimmunity, the thymus does not program your lymphocytes properly, releasing poorly trained T-cells into your bloodstream which attack normal healthy tissues. By balancing your hypothalamus, your thymus does a better job at properly programming your T-cells.

Thyroiditis is not the only type of autoimmune disorder. There are more than eighty types of autoimmune disorders, including lupus, rheumatoid arthritis, multiple sclerosis, hepatitis, celiac disease, pernicious anemia, inflammatory bowel disease, vasculitis, myasthenia gravis, Meniere's disease, Raynaud's phenomenon, chronic fatigue syndrome, and fibromyalgia.

Many autoimmune diseases have similar symptoms, which makes getting a diagnosis frustrating and difficult.

The first symptoms of autoimmunity are often fatigue, muscle aches, and low grade fever - early signs of your body attacking itself. Classically autoimmune diseases are characterized by inflammation, which can cause redness, heat and swelling. But not always. Some autoimmune diseases are internal, like autoimmune thyroiditis, where redness and heat are not seen, while swelling of the thyroid comes later.

Some autoimmune diseases can be diagnosed through blood tests which pick up immune markers like rheumatoid factor for rheumatoid arthritis. Some autoimmune diseases can cause an elevation in ANA – antinuclear antibody – which is a general marker found in the blood that indicates inflammation somewhere in the body. While ANA is not specific and can rise and fall with autoimmune flare-ups and remissions, it is a good starting point if you suspect autoimmunity.

To treat autoimmune flare-ups, conventional medicine prescribes cortisone to reduce inflammation. Chronic use of cortisone can cause significant issues with adrenal function. The adrenal glands make cortisone in response to stress but when you take what you should be making, you hamper your body's ability to make it. Many of my autoimmune patients treated with long-term cortisone have adrenal fatigue. Often untreated autoimmune patients come to me with adrenal issues. Why? Because their exhausted adrenal glands have been working overtime to reduce their autoimmune inflammation.

ELIMINATE THE UNDERLYING TRIGGER OF YOUR AUTOIMMUNITY

It's important to find the deep underlying trigger for each individual's autoimmune disorder. Interestingly enough, the trigger to autoimmune disease is different for everyone. Some autoimmune disorders are triggered by stress. Some by toxins. Some by malnutrition. Some by viruses or intracellular bacterium. Sometimes there are multiple causes that trigger autoimmune response. Often people with one type of autoimmune disease will eventually develop other autoimmune disorders.

It takes some medical detective work to get to the root of autoimmunity. Since each of my patients come with a unique history, I must think out of the box to find what might be causing their autoimmune disorder.

Marsha had longstanding pernicious anemia. For 25 years, she worked long hours as a hair dresser. Beauticians are exposed to many damaging chemicals in their line of work. A mother and grandmother, Marsha got very little sleep, skipped meals, and was exhausted. At 48 years old, she had to have a stent placed in one of her coronary arteries. Her cardiologist could not figure out why Marsha – who's not overweight, has low cholesterol, low blood sugar, and low blood pressure – had a nearly 90% blockage of a main coronary artery.

I suspected a form of autoimmune vasculitis. She responded well to hypothalamic balancing and a novel therapy designed especially for her case. Yet the biggest factor in Marsha's healing was learning to take care of herself.

The thymus lies in your heart chakra. Marsha was attacking herself – autoimmunity – which nearly led to a heart attack. Marsha was like the Tinman who needed a heart. She needed to love herself enough to take care of herself.

You see, most people are really good at taking care of others but not great at taking care of themselves. Especially mothers who tend to put their families' needs over their own. They don't eat properly, don't make time to exercise or meditate or relax. They're so busy taking care of everyone else that they get sick.

When you're on an airplane getting ready to take off, the flight attendant reminds you to put on your oxygen mask before helping others put on theirs. We tend to forget this bit of wisdom.

If you don't take care of yourself, how can you possibly take care of others?

Autoimmunity is the perfect reflection of not putting your oxygen mask on first. And healing this complicated disorder is more than correcting the biochemical imbalances. A shift in attitude is necessary. The sabotaging self-talk must stop. And self-care must begin for healing to happen.

Guess who finally put herself first? Marsha decided to do something she always dreamed of doing. She became a flight attendant! Now she's reminding others to put their oxygen mask on first!

CHAPTER 9

HEALING IN THE DARK

Bob couldn't sleep. In fact, he hadn't had a full night's sleep in over eight years. He tried over-the-counter sleep remedies which would knock him out but never kept him asleep. He would be so exhausted at the end of the day that he would fall asleep right after dinner. He'd find himself an hour or two later on the couch, his wife and children already in bed.

He'd try to go to sleep, but just tossed and turned all night, worried thoughts racing through his mind. If he finally dozed off, his bowels would wake him up between 3 and 5am. Then there was no going back to sleep.

Eight years earlier, Bob had gone through some major financial stress. A high powered executive, he no longer found the energy or motivation to work at the level he used to. Plus, his chronic insomnia was affecting his sex drive and his relationship.

Bob appeared to be the picture of health. A former college athlete, he tried to keep in shape by competing with younger men in the gym. But Bob noticed it was harder to build muscle and he had a soft padding around his midsection.

Bob sighed, "I don't want to admit it, but I think I may need testosterone."

"Bob, I think we'd better start by fixing your gut. It's not normal to have bowel movements in the middle of the night. That's a sign of a dyscircadian rhythm. Until we can get you sleeping through the night and dreaming, you're not going to make enough hormones on your own. You don't want to be taking testosterone for the rest of your life."

Bob just wanted to sleep. So I tentatively offered him Genesis Gold®. "Bob, I'll give you my special formula to reset your circadian rhythm and help you sleep, but you're going to get bloated with gas."

"I don't care. I already have gas and bloating. Please, I just want to sleep."

"I'll give it to you, Bob, but I need you to collect a stool specimen first." He didn't like it, no man does, but Bob was a trooper. He followed my instructions and collected a specimen for a complete digestive stool analysis so we could accurately treat his intestinal dysbiosis. Dysbiosis means your natural bacterial flora is out of balance.

I suspected Bob had an overgrowth of yeast in his gut. While Genesis Gold® provides perfect nutrition for your body, it will also feed Candida. Sure enough, when Bob called in for his blood results, he did have gas, but he actually slept for over five hours and he even had dreams! He was ecstatic! I told him to stop taking Genesis Gold® until I could treat his systemic Candida. Bob wasn't happy but he really wanted to get well.

We treated his Candida so he could absorb all the good stuff in Genesis Gold®. Oh, and he took it in the morning, not at night. I wasn't trying to knock him out – there's lots drugs for that – but to correct his circadian rhythm so he could sleep through the night naturally.

INSOMNIA – THE BANE OF MODERN SOCIETY

Bob's not alone. Over 30% of the population can't sleep either. And it gets worse as you get older. Half the people over the age of 60 complain of insomnia.

Whether you have trouble falling asleep, staying asleep, or both, you have a dyscircadian rhythm.

Insomnia is often initiated by stress. But chronic insomnia is an imbalance of your day/night cycle –your circadian rhythm. Your hypothalamus controls your circadian rhythm. If you can't sleep at night, your hypothalamus is out of balance.

We're all very sensitive to light. Since the introduction of the electric light over one hundred years ago, nearly half of the world is lit up at night. Artificial light disturbs your natural circadian rhythm. If you've ever gone camping, you may have noticed how early you fall asleep.

Without electric lights to keep you up, your body follows the natural day/night cycle.

Your sleep hormone – melatonin – is produced only in the dark. Without adequate melatonin production, your sleep is disturbed, your hormones become imbalanced, and your ability to fight disease is diminished.

Your pineal gland, located in the center of the brain, produces melatonin. Cells in your skin, called chromocytes, carry light wave information to the pineal gland. At dawn, the daylight is a blue wave which stimulates chromocytes to turn off your pineal gland. At dusk, the pink light of sunset blocks the blue rays and your pineal gland begins producing melatonin.

About three hours after dusk, your melatonin production peaks. Melatonin production lasts eight to nine hours in adults, longer in children. At dawn, the drop of melatonin arouses your hypothalamus.

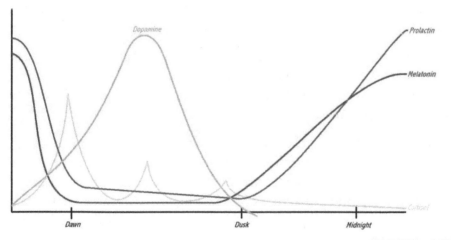

Copyright D Maragopoulos 2016

Once your hypothalamus wakes up, it needs glucose, so it stimulates the adrenal glands to produce cortisol which releases stored sugar. Cortisol stimulates the production of dopamine which is the neurotransmitter of alertness, memory and learning. Dopamine follows natural cortisol rhythms, remaining elevated until mid-afternoon. Schools capitalize on the natural circadian rhythm of this learning hormone by teaching children from 8am to 3pm. The late afternoon slump that makes many of us reach for sugar and caffeine is a reflection of this natural drop in cortisol and dopamine.

Now, teenagers have a different circadian rhythm. Just like infants, teens are in a rapid growth phase and need way more sleep. Their nocturnal hormones do not lower for three hours after dawn. That's why starting school before 9am is not effective for teenagers.

Another extremely important nocturnal hormone is called prolactin. Released by your pituitary gland, prolactin is very high in pregnant and nursing mothers. Its name refers to promoting lactation. In pregnancy, prolactin protects the mother by blocking her cell receptors from the high hormones produced by the fetus. Otherwise, she would grow tumors. After birth, prolactin can protect the mother from conceiving too soon, as long as she is nursing around the clock.

Produced by all ages and both genders, prolactin stimulates your thymus to program your natural killer cells to keep your body free of foreign invaders and cancer. Without sleep, you are prone to disease as your immune system weakens.

Prolactin is produced at high levels at night, peaking about three hours after melatonin peaks and lasting for eight hours. You know you're getting deep sleep when you begin dreaming under the influence of nocturnal prolactin.

If your prolactin production is dyscircadian, meaning it's high during your waking hours rather than at night when you should be asleep, then your lymphocytes are more likely to attack normal healthy cells. High daytime prolactin is like having an active army patrolling while citizens are trying to work. Innocents (your healthy cells) are going to get hurt.

High daytime prolactin not only contributes to autoimmunity, but blocks your steroid hormone receptors.

Take Henry for example:

Henry came to me drug in by his wife. She wanted him to get a thorough check up. He wanted his sex drive back. Otherwise, he claimed to be fine, but he didn't look fine. He had that soft apple-shaped figure and poor muscle tone indicating low testosterone. But what impressed me most was his dazed energy as if he was sleepwalking.

So I checked his testosterone and his prolactin levels. As suspected, his testosterone was really low, low enough to warrant testosterone replacement therapy. But more impressive was his really high prolactin level. Although his levels were not tumor high, just to be safe, I ordered an MRI to rule out a pituitary adenoma.

After I gave him the good news that he did not have a pituitary tumor, I started him on a dopamine agonist to lower his daytime prolactin. He was already noticing more energy and deeper sleep after a couple weeks of taking Genesis Gold®, which was great, but I told him, "Just wait, you're going to get your mojo back within a few weeks."

Sure enough, two months later, his blood tests showed a 50% increase in testosterone! While it was still rather low, he reported a complete turnaround of his libido and sexual performance. That's because now that his prolactin was a healthy daytime low, his testosterone receptors were no longer being blocked. Either way, he's a pretty happy man!

I check an 8-9am serum prolactin on all my patients to see if they are in a healthy circadian rhythm (day-night cycle). Autoimmune patients often have high daytime prolactin. The prolactin level will not necessarily be above the highest range of normal for the patient's gender or age, but anything over 9 after 9am is dyscircadian. Within three hours of dawn, prolactin production is turned off by hypothalamic dopamine. Dopamine allows you to remember your dreams.

In the morning, the blue light waves of the rising sun turn off pineal production of melatonin. Your pineal melatonin cascades into serotonin. A calming hormone, serotonin controls your impulses. And the more serotonin you make during the day, the more melatonin you make at night.

The longer you're in deep REM sleep, the more energy you have during day. That's because your adrenal glands need to rest at night in order to fuel your daytime activity. Adrenal fatigue is a result of chronic insomnia.

TO HEAL YOU MUST SLEEP IN THE DARK

The most significant health information has come from studying nurses. The Nurses Health Studies are the largest and longest running investigations on how lifestyle affects health. Since 1976, nurses have been recruited to study the long-term health consequences of oral contraceptives. Nurses are really good at reporting health and lifestyle issues and the investigators collected much more than they expected.

Data from information collected from nurses over the past forty years shows that those who worked the night shift had higher risk of all disease, including cancer, heart disease, obesity, diabetes, and autoimmune disorders.

Your immune system can't protect you if you don't allow it to work, and it works best when you sleep in the dark.

You've got to go to bed within a few hours of dark to reset your circadian rhythm. I know this is hard, but it's crucial to your health. If you are staying up much past midnight every night, you are missing crucial hours of sleeping in the dark. And you can't make up for it by sleeping in during the daytime.

Although sleep medications are available as temporary relief, they do not promote normal nocturnal hormone production. And without healthy levels of melatonin and prolactin at night, you will not heal.

If you've been staying up past midnight, you can't just go to bed at ten and expect to fall asleep. You must go to bed 15 minutes earlier every few nights. That will slowly reset your nocturnal rhythm so it sticks.

But you have work to do before bed, or you like to watch a few TV shows just to relax. Remember the blue light from the computer and television screens suppresses your melatonin production. That's why you have trouble falling asleep. You are actually getting a second wind after dark by exposing yourself to the daytime light waves coming from your TV and computer screen.

If you must expose yourself after dark to a computer, television, iPad, smart phone, or other electronic devices, then use pink-tinted sunglasses to mimic the dusk and increase your nighttime melatonin and prolactin levels. I know they look weird, but pink glasses work. Just don't make a habit of being on the computer after dark.

And do NOT go to sleep with the TV on. Televisions in bedrooms are one of the prime reasons people suffer from insomnia. Plus, all the digital lights flashing in your bedroom are disturbing your sleep. Cover them at night.

But you say you cover your eyes with nightshades. Let me tell you about a sleep study that was done on college students.

College students will do anything for money. So the researchers kept them up until they were exhausted, then had them go to sleep in a completely dark room. Without waking them up, the researchers measured the students' salivary melatonin levels which were high because the students were sleeping in the dark.

Then the researchers shined a pen light on the back of the students' knees. And their salivary melatonin levels bottomed out. That tiny spot of light was all it took to disturb their sleep.

So NO light in your bedroom at all.

BALANCE YOUR HYPOTHALAMUS TO RESET YOUR CIRCADIAN RHYTHM

I really did not appreciate how the hypothalamus affects our sleep cycles until I created Genesis Gold®.

You see, I suffered from somnambulism, or sleep walking, for eighteen years. Rarely did I get a restful night's sleep. Most nights I slept less than four or five hours. Many nights I found myself outside clutching a pillow. Kind of scary and definitely not good for my health. I managed my days by running on fumes, exercising obsessively, and eating way too much sugar.

Then I created Genesis Gold®, and within three weeks, I began sleeping through the night. My sugar cravings stopped and I didn't need to exercise like a maniac to stay sane. In fact, for the first few months, I slept over ten hours a night – my body trying to catch up from years of lack of sleep.

Balancing the hypothalamus takes time to reset the circadian rhythm, so Genesis Gold® is not an immediate sleep aide, but instead gets to the core issue, balancing the brain chemistry, restoring optimal hypothalamic functioning, and, in time, deepening and lengthening your sleep cycles.

CHAPTER 10

BELIEF BECOMES

Nina was sent to me for a psycho-spiritual healing. She had advanced stage IV head and neck cancer and there was nothing medicine could do for her. A lovely blond woman in her late forties, Nina sat quietly before me, a cupcake sized tumor protruding from her neck. I took her hands in mine.

"Nina, if you are finished here on earth, I'll help you transition. If you're not ready to die, I'll help you live. It's your choice."

Tearing up, she smiled at me, "I'm not ready to die."

"Ok. Then we've got some work to do."

Conventional therapy of radical surgery and radiation would have given her a few years, but a very poor quality of life – inability to eat, to speak, to hear, facial paralysis and blindness. Nina chose an alternative route. Without much hope for her advanced cancer since her diagnosis, Nina exhausted all the complementary cancer treatments she could on her own.

What Nina hadn't explored was the psycho-spiritual root of her dis-ease. It became clear to me during our first two-hour consult that Nina had planted a death wish a long time ago and it was related to her mother.

"What happened when your mother died?"

Nina admitted to being so devastated at the death of her beloved mother some 20 years earlier that she just wanted to die, too. But Nina had a young daughter of her own, so she stayed. But she never got over her grief. And that death seed got planted deep in her subconscious just waiting to blossom.

Now, of course, there were other things that contributed to Nina's cancer. She smoked in her youth. Her diet wasn't great. She was exposed to heavy metals in her line of work. And her mother did die of breast cancer.

Yet how many people have all these exposures and live long, disease free lives. Is it good genes? Or is it an attitude?

Belief becomes. We manifest what we believe. If we believe we will die young, age like our parents, get the same diseases as they did, then we probably will. And if we live their same lifestyle, then it's even more likely we will succumb to the family curse – be it cancer, heart disease, Alzheimer's.

You can change your destiny through your lifestyle choices and your beliefs.

My work with Nina was to explore her beliefs that seeded her vulnerability to cancer and to find out what she had to live for. Nina really wanted to live long enough to see her daughter graduate from college and get married.

So I helped Nina have the highest quality life possible. She faithfully did all her homework. Yes, I give my patients homework – things to read, to meditate on, affirmations, lifestyle changes.

Nina attended her daughter's college graduation, and then a year later danced at her daughter's wedding. And when she had completed these goals, Nina was done. I then spent time helping her family let her go. She died peacefully at home nearly five years after we first met, some seven years longer than the doctors originally gave her.

Nina's daughter is still one of my sweetest patients. The same age as my children, she's open to my maternal love and advice. They all feel like family to me. Full Circle Family Health has provided me the space to help my patients from birth to death. It's a privilege to heal body, mind, and soul.

UNVEIL THE CORE BELIEF THAT MAY BE CAUSING YOUR DISEASE

This is the hardest part of the treatment. Finding what may be underlying my patient's dis-ease at a psycho-spiritual level takes some finesse. Thankfully, balancing their hypothalamus with Genesis Gold® can deepen their sleep, and often their subconscious reveals the truth to them in dreams.

As I get to know a patient, their core issue becomes apparent, and when they are ready to deal with it, we do. Sometimes I am blessed to have a new patient come to me for a consult and they are so ripe (ready to heal) that I can "see" what their core issue is, speak it, and the patient says, "Yes, that makes sense!"   Healing is much faster when we deal with the psycho-spiritual along with the physical.

Dis-ease is your body's way of talking to you. I'd rather your body whisper than scream what it needs. That's why I created Genesis Gold®, to help us know more clearly what our bodies need to be optimally well. I call it becoming innate.

OVER THE RAINBOW

Like DOROTHY in the <u>Wizard of Oz</u>, we are all on our healing journey, wishing for health that we believe is just over the rainbow. A major health crisis becomes the tornado that takes us from our old life to a new healthy way of being.

We are blessed to have our intuition, like a **GOOD WITCH**, to guide us. Along the **YELLOW BRICK ROAD** of healing, we learn to optimize our brain function (**SCARECROW**), strengthen our immunity (**TINMAN**), and gain courage (**COWARDLY LION**) as our hormones come into harmony. Then we face our fears and doubts that seem determined to sabotage our progress like the **WICKED WITCH.**

So you might dissolve your fears like water dissolved the wicked witch, the time is ripe to unveil the emotional roots of your health issues.

Remember in Chapter 2, I aligned your seven endocrine glands with the seven power points, called chakras, in your body? The chakras correspond to the seven colors of the rainbow. From red to violet, from root to crown, energy flows. Energy is the base of the DMAR® Pyramid of Health.

When these energy centers are blocked, the corresponding hormones become imbalanced.

Here's my chakra lady to illustrate the seven chakras and endocrine glands.

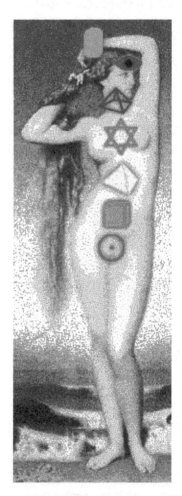

- Your 1st root chakra corresponds with your gonads – ovaries or testes. The color is **RED** and the energy is about survival. The purpose of your gonads is to procreate, to pass your DNA on to the next generation. You do not have to have children to fulfill your creative energy. Any creative endeavor – art, music, design, gardening, creating your new life – fulfills this chakra's purpose. If your creative energies are blocked, you may develop issues in your reproductive organs.

Gus loved the dramatic arts. A teacher by profession, he loved directing plays. When he began to manage his partner's business, there was little time to pursue his art. Gus came to me with a large inflamed prostate that had

Copyright D Maragopoulos 2016

not responded to conventional therapy. I offered him alternative remedies, but the biggest breakthrough for Gus was when he understood that his inflamed prostate was his body's way of communicating with him. Once he started making time to express himself creatively, his prostatitis began to heal.

- Your 2nd navel chakra corresponds with your pancreas. The color is **ORANGE** and the energy is about pleasure. I call it being open to receive the sweetness of life. The purpose of your pancreas is to get sugar into your cells so you have the energy to create your best life. Think of this chakra as the energetic fuel for survival. Diabetes and insulin resistance are the ultimate blockage to receiving the sweetness of life.

Patricia had high blood pressure, high cholesterol, diabetes, and could not lose weight. She came to me for nutritional counseling and alternative therapies to control her blood sugar and cholesterol. Patricia lived with an alcoholic husband. For years I counseled her regarding how to eat, exercise, and release her codependency with her spouse. I wish I had a vat of transdermal hormones big enough to heal her life. But until Patricia could be open to change, she battled her diseases.

Within a few months of starting Genesis Gold®, a shift happened for Patricia. She began to see the good in her life. She began speaking positively about herself. She began taking better care of herself. She finally realized that she had to put on her oxygen mask first. And when her husband saw the change in her, he became open to help. For the first time, he stuck with a sober living plan. When Patricia was finally open to receive the sweetness in life, she was no longer insulin resistant. Her diabetes resolved itself. But more so, Patricia was happy.

- Your 3rd solar plexus chakra corresponds with your adrenal glands. The color is **YELLOW** and the energy is about power. Your adrenal glands control your stress response, how you physically and emotionally deal with what's happening in your life, how you either maintain your personal power or give it away.

Remember Sally who suffered with hair loss? Her hair loss was related to her adrenal function. Her excessive DHEA converted to testosterone and knocked out her hair follicles. And then after years of high stress, her adrenals became so fatigued, she didn't make enough hormones to grow healthy hair. Sally gave away her power to the men in her life, from her father to her boyfriends to her husband. While chelation cleared her blocked receptor sites and Genesis Gold® provided the nutrition to heal her hormonal imbalance, Sally's hair returned to its former glory when she finally stopped giving away her power.

- Your 4th heart chakra corresponds with your thymus. The color is **GREEN** and the energy is about compassion for self and others. Are you protecting yourself with a strong immune system? Or are you attacking yourself with an autoimmune condition? Having compassion for yourself is the first step to healing an imbalanced immune system.

  Carrie came to me with crippling Rheumatoid Arthritis. She hated the side effects of conventional therapy. I worked with her for years helping her make the necessary lifestyle changes and providing the proper micronutrients to heal her condition. Unfortunately, Carrie felt victimized by her life, by her disease. She berated herself for her inability to function as she once had. Over time, she learned that healing began with loving herself. When she was compassionate to herself, she took great care of herself and her Rheumatoid Arthritis would go into remission. When she spoke lovingly about herself, her life, even her disease, she would be pain free and functional.

- Your 5th throat chakra corresponds with your thyroid. The color is **BLUE** and the energy is about expressing your truth. Speaking our truth can be difficult. Sometimes we don't even know what our truth is. When we have difficulty expressing ourselves, we cannot live our most authentic lives. We live our lives for others, feeling unfulfilled, unheard. Sometimes even those closest to you do not know the real you.

Abigail suffered from hyperthyroidism. The medications given to her to reverse her disease knocked her thyroid out, so after years of being rail thin and manic, she now was overweight and depressed. Abigail had lost herself. She hid the love of her life from her family who could not accept her sexual preferences. She worked at a job she hated rather than pursuing her passion in the fine arts. Abigail was afraid to speak her truth. Helping Abigail see how she was not being true to herself was the first step in healing her thyroid disorder. As Genesis Gold® helped her sleep more deeply, she practiced in her dreams speaking her truth. The increased energy and elevated mood she experienced helped Abigail start living a more authentic life and her thyroid disorder began to heal.

- Your 6th third eye chakra corresponds with your pituitary gland. The color is **INDIGO** and the energy is about having clear insight. Being able to know yourself and why you are going through a particular life event requires an unblocked third eye. It's easy to see what others' life lessons are. It's more difficult to see our own.

Giovanni had impossibly big feet and hands for his stature. Only five six, he wore a size 13 shoe. I told him he needed to get his pituitary gland checked. Not until he developed excruciating headaches did he finally follow my advice. The MRI showed a large pituitary tumor. Surgery to remove the tumor relieved the headaches but did not fix his unhappy marriage. Giovanni prided himself on advising other men about their relationships, yet did not have the insight to heal his own.

- Your 7th crown chakra corresponds with your pineal gland. The color is **VIOLET** and the energy is about your connection to the divine. In many cultures, one prays with a bowed head, the crown of the head open to receive divine guidance. Dreamtime is often the most open we are to that small still voice of divine wisdom.

Susan suffered from chronic insomnia. Her salivary melatonin levels were nonexistent. She felt disconnected and had very little appreciation for the wonder of life. She was just too tired. In spite of turning off all her lights at night, trying to go to bed at a decent hour, supplements to knock her out and stay asleep, Susan could not sleep. When she finally started taking Genesis Gold®, she slept for the first time in years, but nightmares disturbed her. It was clear to me that Susan had a lot to work out at the subconscious level so I asked her to keep a dream journal. With some guidance, she began to make sense of her dreams. Once she cleared her subconscious of all the pain she feared to face, Susan became open to meditation. With healthy circadian rhythms, Susan receives guidance through prayerful meditation during the day and sweet dreams at night.

HEALER HEAL THYSELF

A heavily laden fog dripped down my mare's legs as she pranced excitedly beneath me. Holding the slick reins in check, I hesitated at the crest of the trail. Steep, wet asphalt lay before us and I had a flash of premonition – I saw my mare fall, trapping me beneath her. Well aware that thought creates reality, I tried to clear my mind and rode on.

Not fifty yards later, my mare spooked. In an effort to stop her from bolting, I turned her up the sharp grade. She slipped and, as if rehearsed, I vaulted off her back. Thankfully, not pinned under a thousand pounds of terrified horse, I did manage to save my skull from what would have been a concussive blow. Unfortunately, I landed squarely on my mouth. Scrambling to my feet, I ran after her, touching my bloodied lip to extract my front teeth.

With the help of a kind gardener, I caught my runaway horse and made it home. I tended to her wounds first, my teeth in my pocket. Typical of most healers, I am reluctant to ask for help. Thankfully, my sleeping husband perceived my unspoken distress. He worked the graveyard shift but jumped out of bed to drive me to the emergency dentist.

The dentist shook his head when I handed him the cup of milk in which my broken teeth floated. "I cannot replace these..."

I tried to encourage him, "I know you can do it. Please, you must believe in your ability."

While I prayed, focusing on the living essence of my teeth with healing intentions, he performed the procedure, and then made me promise to go to the emergency room for x-rays. Although I did everything the dentist recommended as well as all the holistic remedies I would have prescribed for someone with similar injuries, I bemoaned my ill fortune.

My face was a mess – my nose, lips and chin skinned, swollen and bruised, like I had been beaten. I called my sister, who cried, "Oh, Deb, your beautiful teeth!" No braces, no cavities, straight and strong, my vanity lay in the perfection of my teeth. How could this have happened? I taught my patients that everything happens for a reason, but I couldn't see why. I even called my spiritual mentor, who provided only practical advice. I was on my own.

I believe each of the seven chakras of the body deliver purposeful messages, so what was my fifth chakra, which represents speaking my truth, saying? I fell asleep wondering and awoke Saturday at dawn to meditate in nature.

Surrounded by my animals, even my very sore but sorry mare, I sat at the edge of a huge, ugly gaping hole. We had just moved into the country and, having lived through one unbearably hot summer, began construction on a swimming pool. Our land was scarred and so was I. My mare nuzzled my back, while the dogs whined piteously with me.

Suddenly, I heard a voice. Not that small quiet voice that compassionately guides, but one so obnoxious that the animals gave me a wide berth.

Stop feeling sorry for yourself. You've been given a gift...practice what you preach and heal yourself.

My smile cracked my newly scabbed lips. This accident was a gift! Hugging my horse, I thanked her. Have you ever seen a horse smile? Remember Mr. Ed showing his big teeth? Well, that's what she did, smiled at my recognition of her part on my soul's path.

I then hurried into the house and took a good look in the mirror. Instead of seeing a broken reflection, I saw the healing. I became my own best cheerleader. I told my body what a great job it was doing every time I washed my wounds. I blessed every herbal supplement for helping my system recover. Every ounce, I drank in gratitude (dentist's orders – no solid foods) praying that each nutrient find its way to repair the damage.

And by Monday, I was whole and healed, not a single scar. A couple of days later, I went back to the emergency room to pick up some x-rays and the nurses didn't recognize me. Oh, yes, and to the dentist's great surprise, my teeth took root.

Healing is an innate power within each and every one of us. It is encoded, I believe, in the unexpressed DNA, ready to be turned on by the power of our intentions.

As a healer, I have learned that I do not heal anyone, but educate them to heal themselves. I provide biochemical and psycho-spiritual counsel. I hold the intention, the energy of health and well-being mirrored in my body, in my DNA.

Once a young woman I had been seeing since her teens insisted on an office exam just six months after her annual pap smear. There was no medical reason for her to come, so I questioned her. She very eloquently answered, "I just need to sit in your presence, feel your vibration, and I am set for about a half-year."

I have a dear older patient who makes me promise after every visit, every phone call, to stay well. "We need your vibrancy to remember how to be whole."

After working all my life to be an example of health through exercise, nutrition, and lifestyle choices, I know that my true talent is in perceiving every event in my life as a lesson. Plus, a positive attitude can be seriously protective.

Once in Seattle, I attended a detoxification seminar. After the morning presentations about all the toxins in our everyday environment, we were released for lunch. This group of holistic nurses, physicians, naturopaths and chiropractors hesitated to choose anything from the menu of what seemed to be a reasonably healthy restaurant.

With my usual gusto, I ordered tuna on fire, and the rest of them looked at me like I was nuts. One woman asked if I had paid attention to the statistics on heavy metal contamination of fatty fish.

"Why, yes. I took scrupulous notes, but I do not believe in my vulnerability to toxicity. At this very moment your fear is sucking the mercury right out of my tuna."

I have eaten contaminated seafood all my life, yet do not test positive for heavy metal toxicity. Is it favorable genetics, perhaps...or my attitude?

Whenever I see a sick, contagious patient, I say to myself, "This is not your bug!" and rarely catch their illness. When I do become ill, it is usually a psycho-spiritual dilemma in which I have been paying little attention and finally my body is reminding me to take care of it.

My accident was truly a gift. I had never been seriously injured before in spite of vigorous and dangerous activities – mountain biking, skiing, scuba diving, road bike racing – never gave myself a chance to learn how healing works.

What I learned was this: That gratitude is the key to the power of intention. With all the positive encouragement, my body rapidly responded. It makes me wonder how much faster I might have healed if I hadn't spent the first day fussing over my predicament. Fear definitely hampers healing.

Mind over matter? I have seen, over and over again, patients worrying themselves into disease...yet I have also seen the power of hope, love and gratitude to cure what was deemed incurable.

In my experience, most of my breast cancer patients tend to take care of everyone but themselves. Unless they receive that lesson, they do not survive the disease. I have some amazing women in my practice who have healed themselves by understanding that their cancer was their souls' cry for help, not attending to their soul's need for so long that their body had to get their attention. Some use traditional allopathic treatments, others use only natural therapies, most who seek my care combine the two. I do not dictate to them what they must do to heal, what therapeutics to choose, but counsel them to make peace with their bodies, find the gift in their disease, and begin healing with the faith that they have the innate ability to cure themselves.

The spring following my accident, I attended a Science and Consciousness conference in Albuquerque and realized how I had healed myself. That year, Gregg Braden spoke on the Isaiah Effect, which illustrated how prayer and healing worked through clear intention fueled by loving gratitude. So with my experience and the equation for manifestation, I began teaching my patients. Sometimes the Isaiah Effect worked, but not always, especially in dealing with relationship issues.

The next year, while writing my first novel, <u>LoveDance</u>, I had an epiphany. The two-part equation was missing a factor! I have always struggled with duality in any way. This reality is not black and white, but a rainbow of possibilities. I am not the only soul in the universe, but am part of a great whole. When my intentions do not become manifest as rapidly as I desire, my husband reminds me that it's not in Deborah-timing, but Divine-timing.

In researching my novel, I discovered Neil Douglas Klotz. His work explained that the terms translated as good and evil from the Aramaic – tava and bisha – actually meant ripe and unripe. So Divine-timing meant Ripe timing.

The Isaiah Effect was missing an element.

It was not $X + Y$ = manifestation but $X + Y + Z$ = manifestation, where X = clear intention, Y = pure desire, and Z = ripe timing.

So now I counsel my patients to continue to hold clear intentions of healing their bodies, their minds, their relationships. Fuel their intentions, not with fear, but with loving gratitude. And in ripe timing, they will manifest, and the rewards will be sweet indeed.

Every day, I thank my body for her strength, her health, her vitality. Like taking my Genesis Gold®, sleeping in the dark, and eating locally grown organic foods, I see gratitude as a proactive means to support my wellbeing. I am trying very hard to practice what I preach, so neither my body nor my inner voice must scream to get my attention. And thankfully, now that guiding voice has become a gentle whisper.

CHAPTER 11

YOUR NUTRITIONAL PATH TO WELLNESS

Nutrition is the key. You are what you eat. Your hormones, your neurotransmitters, your cytokines are a reflection of your nutritional intake. To heal your body, you need to eat a balanced diet. And your diet should match your DNA.

While there's not One Diet for Every Body, the great thing about optimizing your genetic expression with Genesis Gold® is that you will "know" exactly what your body needs. You will become your own body whisperer. You will crave what your body needs.

Every winter I used to suffer from Seasonal Affective Disorder. When the nights get longer with less sun exposure, you make less serotonin and dopamine. You become sad. You crave carbohydrates. Some people gain a lot of weight. I would get anxious, moody, and yes, sad. For me, the sad time hits when we have to change the clocks back in the fall.

Well, the year I started taking Genesis Gold® about two weeks before we changed the clocks back, I began craving orange vegetables – pumpkin, butternut squash, yams. I couldn't get enough. And for the first time, I didn't have seasonal affective disorder. My body was talking to me. "Hey, the days are getting shorter. Eat squash – the brighter orange, the better."

DMAR® NUTRITIONAL PATH TO WELLNESS

Until you become attuned to your body, I created my DMAR® Nutritional Path to Wellness to help you make the best food choices for your body.

My DMAR® Nutritional Path to Wellness is based upon the Mediterranean Diet. Not just because I'm Italian (Maragopoulos is

Greek), but because the Mediterranean Diet has been shown in studies to be the healthiest for the majority of people. It's plant based, low glycemic, and provides moderate amounts of good fats and adequate protein. That combination is best for hormone production.

The basis of my DMAR® Nutritional Path to Wellness is: If nature makes it, you can eat it.

Eat locally grown organic produce in season and naturally raised animal products for the highest level of nutrition and lowest level of toxins. Drink pure filtered water. Avoid processed foods.

It's simple. Give your body the highest quality foods and your body will give you its very best.

Here are the four cornerstones of my DMAR® Nutritional Path to Wellness:

1. Protein - your basic building blocks

Protein provides the necessary essential amino acids for hormone production, healthy brain chemistry and proper immune function. Adequate protein intake is essential for proper hypothalamic functioning. Animal protein provides all the essential amino acids you need to make a new you.

Hold on! Am I telling you that you have to eat meat to be healthy? Not necessarily. But you'd better be an excellent vegetarian to get enough protein to make enough neurotransmitters, hormones, and immune factors for your omnivorous human body.

For seven years, I was a vegetarian. A really educated vegetarian and a gourmet cook, I knew exactly how to combine plants to get protein in my diet. Plus, there were lots of vegetarian protein alternative foods to make complete meals for my family.

Then I began taking Genesis Gold®. Within in a few weeks, I was craving meat. Yes, craving! Like chocolate. I was dreaming about rotisserie chicken. Nothing satisfied me. I felt guilty. My whole family followed me into a vegetarian lifestyle and now all I could think about was eating animals!

When I began the research on Genesis Gold®, I decided to join my research subjects and stop everything else I was taking – vitamins, minerals, and herbs to support my adrenals; amino acids to balance my brain chemistry; bioidentical hormones and the supplements to metabolize and detoxify them – and I decided to listen to my body.

My body wanted animal protein. So I got a rotisserie chicken and ate the whole thing! Holy moly! I had never eaten that much meat at one time in my life. In fact, I didn't even like meat. If someone was eating rare red meat near me, I felt sick. Yet during both of my pregnancies, I craved rare meat. "Bloody for your blood," as Cher's character from the movie Moonstruck says.

I checked my own blood levels and found I was anemic. Eating animal protein quickly raised my hemoglobin. The myoglobin in rare red meat would have been better, but the chicken did the trick. The problem was my husband could smell it on me. When I came clean, he gladly gave up vegetarianism for the diet of his ancestors. Greek boys are taught at a young age how to roast lamb. Steve is Mr. BBQ. There's not much he can't cook over an open fire. The problem is he does such an amazing job grilling meat, fish, and vegetables, well, it's hard to eat out.

So I say, "Listen to your body!"

If you are vegetarian for health reasons, it may not be the healthiest diet for you. It's like the Asian diet – rich in soy. Great if you're Asian. If not, all that soy will negatively affect your thyroid function.

Your DNA needs what your ancestors ate, how they ate it, and how they lived.

2.   Fat – for the health of your cells

My ancestors ate a lot of fat – way more than I did as a vegetarian. When I was about 30, I was competing in triathlons – swimming, cycling and running. I was lean, really lean, about 12% body fat, although I weighed more then since bone and muscle weigh more than fat. Anyhow, I was eating a low fat, low protein, carb-based diet. Back then, carb loading was all the rage in competitive long-distant athletics. But I was burning so much energy with all that activity that I was hungry **ALL THE TIME!** I couldn't get enough calories and craved sugar.

At my annual physical, my internist reported that my cholesterol was great – only 130! I was appalled. My HDL was less than 25. That's not healthy. You can't make hormones without cholesterol, and with such a low HDL, I had no cardiovascular protection.

I decided right then and there to give up my low fat diet and eat like my ancestors did. Lots and lots of olive oil. We practically drink it! We put it on everything. Studies have shown that vegetables roasted with olive oil retain their nutrients. No other oil compares.

I started eating whole fat everything. No more nonfat, low fat stuff. Whole fat yogurt. Real butter. Real cheese. Whole eggs. Still no meat, yet. This is before Genesis Gold® and I'm still a vegetarian.

Guess what? In just a few months, my cholesterol rose to 180 with an HDL of 90. Now that's fantastic. Your HDL should make up at least one third of your total cholesterol. Remember, this was before we measured cholesterol particle size.

Oh, and my hair and my skin were much, much healthier. Plus, my sugar cravings nearly disappeared. I say nearly, because PMS has a mind of her own, and that time of the month, well, let's just say you'd better not get between me and chocolate.

So bottom line: Fats are great. Not transfats. Avoid those. Transfats are manmade fats like hydrogenated oils. Transfats are not healthy fats. Studies have shown that diets rich in transfats increase the risk of cancer, heart disease, diabetes, immune disorders, and learning disabilities. This is one of the many reasons the Standard American Diet is deservedly known as SAD.

Healthy hormone function requires healthy fat consumption. If you don't eat enough fat, your hormones cannot get into your cells.

Cell membranes are like a butter sandwich, made up of two layers of glycoproteins (the bread) with phospholipids in between (the butter). Within the butter imagine olives – little doorways that allow hormones into cells. These hormone receptor sites require essential fatty acids for healthy function.

Fats provide essential fatty acids known as Omega-3s, Omega-6s, Omega-9s. The goal is to get more Omega-3s than Omega-6s and Omega-9s. Seafood is rich in Omega-3s.

Healthy fat consumption begins in utero. In the last trimester of pregnancy, the fetus gets bathed in a type of Omega-3s called docosahexaenoic acid. DHA is crucial for neurological development, visual acuity, and cognition. Because of the Standard American Diet, most American women do not eat enough seaweeds and fish to have adequate DHA available for their unborn children, nor enough to supply in their breast milk.

Babies born to women who do not consume enough healthy fat, specifically DHA, have a higher risk of developmental delays and learning disabilities. I believe that was what happened with my first child.

Being an American teenager in the 1970s, I ate very little fat. Fat was the enemy. Fat made you fat. Medical science told us high fat diets caused heart disease and obesity. We all believed it. So by the time I became pregnant, I had no healthy fat stores. That probably contributed to my toxemia and premature delivery. It definitely contributed to Jarys' ADHD.

When Jarys was eight, he asked me to take him to a brain doctor. He couldn't concentrate like the rest of the kids. The psychologist who specialized in learning disabled children interviewed Jarys, his teachers, and us. He couldn't find any evidence of a learning disability. Granted, Jarys was reading at the age of three. He was so well read by the third grade that you couldn't play Trivial Pursuit with the kid!

Jarys asked Dr. Mick to give him the video game test. Dr. Mick was floored. He was part of a research team that was beta-testing a video game to determine attention deficits. I told you this kid knew things. Must have been all those female hormones in utero bathing his brain. Jarys tested off the charts for ADHD.

I researched everything possible to help Jarys. One of the most effective things we did was add fatty fish into his diet. The omega-3s provided by seafood helped him tremendously. Yet until I created

Genesis Gold®, Jarys needed a small dose of ADHD drugs on school days. He hasn't needed them since.

Fats are essential for healthy cell membranes, hormone production, and neurotransmitter function. Eating healthy fats helps you feel satiated by slowing down the exit time of the food from your stomach. Listen to your body, it will tell you when it's had enough.

Low fat diets with poor quality proteins are a recipe for hormonal dysfunction leading to hypothalamic-pituitary imbalance.

How much fat do you need? I suggest 30% of your calories come from fat and one-third of all your fats should be saturated. Animal fats are saturated fats. The rest of your fats should come from plant sources – nuts, seeds, coconut, olives, avocados, olive oil.

3. Carbohydrates – a plant based diet

In spite of all that animal protein and healthy fats, the majority of my diet is plants – lots and lots of vegetables. The Mediterranean Diet is rich with vegetables. Easily 2/3 of my plate is covered with lots of colorful vegetables. Very few people get enough vegetables in their diet, and if they do there's usually very little variety. They eat the same few veggies day in and day out – mostly salads because most people don't know how to cook vegetables.

One of my favorite ways to cook vegetables is to roast them in olive oil. Remember, olive oil retains the nutrients in vegetables. There aren't many vegetables that can't be roasted – asparagus, beets, broccoli, carrots, cauliflower, fennel, garlic, onions, winter squash, yams and my favorite – brussel sprouts! Don't tell me you don't like brussel sprouts until you've tasted them roasted.

Now, greens need to be sautéed. Dandelion, mustard, beet, collard greens. Spinach, kale, chard. Sauté in olive oil over medium heat just until the leaves turn bright green, and then squeeze a little lemon juice on them so your body can absorb the minerals from the greens.

Forget boiling or steaming your vegetables. You're losing all the nutrients. Plus, they're mushy!

What about salads?

I love salads but you can't absorb iron from raw greens no matter how much olive oil you dress them in. Salads are roughage, providing fiber so you can move your bowels. Add roasted veggies into your salads, some protein – like nuts, seeds, cheese, eggs, leftover meat, poultry or fish – and avocado or olives for healthy fat. And forget bottled dressing. Olive oil, vinegar or juice, a little pepper, sea salt, a sprinkle of herbs, that's all you need for a well-dressed salad.

What about fruit?

Fruit is great – if it's locally grown, freshly picked, and organic. Eat all you want. Don't worry, Mother Nature made sure you can only eat so much fruit. If you eat too much, it goes right through you. I remember as a kid climbing into our neighbor's plum tree and eating all the ripe plums I could get my little hands on. Oh, yes, you guessed it. My tummy would ache and I would have the runs. Too much fruit.

Forget fruit juice. A splash to flavor water or to mix your Genesis Gold® in, that's fine. Otherwise you're drinking too much sugar.

What about grains?

Whole grains are great. Unfortunately, most people eat too much of them. Grains are complex carbohydrates made up of starches which are really long chains of sugar. Starches are really easy to digest and absorb. The outdated food pyramid derived most of its calories from grains. Unless you're going to burn off all those starchy carb calories, you're going to store them as body fat.

SAD is the Standard American Diet. It's very SAD and the basis of most of our health issues. It's chemically laden with pesticides, herbicides, dyes, and artificial ingredients. There's too much sugar, too much starch, too many transfats. There's not enough healthy fat and not nearly enough vegetables!

Most American restaurants are SAD. They serve one or two portions of starch – potatoes, pasta, rice – plus a basket of bread. Maybe a little bit of veggies, but very little. The starchy carbs and the meat take up most the plate.

Some of my patients don't get it. I'll put them on my Insulin Resistant Diet which is just vegetables, protein and fats. And they ask, "What about whole wheat pasta?" No, no starches. "Well, what about brown rice?" No, no starches. "Ok, I'm not eating bread anymore," they say, "maybe an occasional tortilla." No tortillas. That's starch.

It's hard. They grew up on the food pyramid that is grain based. We were taught to fill up on starches. And look how obese America is now. Don't even get me started on high fructose corn syrup!

My Italian American family thought I had gone to the dark side when I became a health nut. "Flour and sugar are the bane of society" was my battle cry. I still believe it, but I'm not so radical.

Everything in moderation. I eat sugar, just not that often. I bake for the holidays and I eat what I make, but afterwards follow my Insulin Resistant Diet so my weight doesn't yo-yo. Constantly losing and gaining weight is really bad for your hypothalamus. Your hypothalamus will set your weight set point higher every time you crash diet. So be sensible.

Avoid sugar and chemicals and limit starchy carbohydrates. This enables your cells to reopen insulin receptors and reverse insulin resistance. As your metabolism repairs, muscle and bone builds and your body requires fuel.

You should eat when you're hungry, but make sure that you eat proteins and fats, non-starchy vegetables and natural carbohydrates (not manmade). Carbohydrates that are quickly broken down to glucose, like sugars and starches, have the highest glycemic level. When you eat fewer carbohydrates and more healthy proteins and fats, your insulin levels stay lower, and glucagon – the fat mobilizing hormone – is produced to allow your body to break down its fat stores to use as energy.

What if you're overweight?

The secret is to eat less carb calories than you expend. I know calories are calories, but your body can easily break down carbohydrates into glucose. It takes much more work (energy and enzymes) to break down fats and proteins into glucose for energy. If you exercise a few times a week **AND** consume fewer carbohydrate calories, you force your body to go into your fat storage for energy.

Now your weight will not change right away – fat weighs much less than lean body mass (muscle and bone) – but you will lose inches as your body composition shifts.

Another secret is to consume **NO CARBS** after 4 PM. That does not include non-starchy vegetables. Between 3-5 PM, your adrenals take a siesta. You will crave carbs, but avoiding them will force your body to use its stored sugar.

Carbohydrates are energy foods. You do not have to count non-starchy vegetables because they are low glycemic index foods (they do not easily convert into sugar). You must count all the rest –starches, fruits and starchy vegetables. Avoid white flour, white sugar and highly refined foods.

It's simple math. To lose weight, you must take in fewer calories than you expend. Carbohydrate calories are more easily stored as body fat. So a diet low in carbs, rich in healthy fats and protein with lots of colorful vegetables is best to reverse insulin resistance.

It does take time for the hypothalamus to come into balance as your body heals. Reproductive hormones are the last to balance. Reversal of insulin resistance, along with adrenal and thyroid regulation comes first as the hypothalamic-pituitary axis corrects. Your mood improves early, reflecting increased endorphin production. Remember, Genesis Gold® balances your hypothalamus. And your hypothalamus controls your metabolism and your weight set point.

As your hypothalamus readjusts to a healthier state, you will notice a healthier weight set point.

The secret to my DMAR® Nutritional Path to Wellness is figuring out how much protein and carbohydrates you need based on your body composition and activity level. My DMAR® Nutritional Path to Wellness includes formulas to figure out your exact macronutrient need. Macronutrients are proteins, fats, and carbohydrates. Micronutrients are vitamins, minerals, and cofactors.

THE DIET WARS

I don't like the word diet. I don't like to tell my patients exactly what to eat. I would rather teach them how to eat – what's healthy, what's not, how to prepare food for the greatest nutritional benefit.

Plus, diets are used to lose weight. I prefer a nutritional plan. But I understand that some people need more guidance. They want to know exactly what to eat for breakfast, lunch and dinner. So for my overweight patients and those with high cholesterol, diabetes, or insulin resistance, I developed my Insulin Resistant Diet.

It's basically my DMAR® Nutritional Path to Wellness without any grains, starchy vegetables, or fruit – and of course, no sugar. My Insulin Resistant Diet tells you exactly what and how much to consume to reverse your insulin resistance and lose body fat.

Sometimes you need to clean out your liver before starting my Insulin Resistant Diet. If your lifestyle is toxic – lots of stress, traveling, poor food choices, no sleep – I developed a dietary Liver Cleanse that works great to clear out toxins. I follow it twice a year for three days – after indulging during the holidays and at the beginning of summer. And once a week, we eat what I call a Liver Cleanse dinner. It's kept my husband, who tends towards gallbladder issues, healthy. My patients love it as a simple way to clean up their bodies using lots of veggies!

You can download my DMAR® Nutritional Path to Wellness, my Liver Cleanse, and my Insulin Resistant Diet at www.thehormonequeen.com/gifts

Very few of my patients follow the Standard American Diet. Most of them have educated themselves and have tried all types of alternative nutritional plans – the paleo diet, raw foods, the GAPS diet. They come to me because, in spite of their best attempts, they aren't healthy. That's where Genesis Gold® comes in to heal their biochemistry and help them know what they need to eat to be optimally well.

4. Water – the most essential nutrient

Water is the stuff of life. Every living thing needs water. You need at least ½ ounce of water per pound of body weight (30ml/kilo) every day.

Start by drinking a big glass of water in the morning. Your hydration meter within your hypothalamus will then trigger your thirst for the rest of the day.

What if you're just not thirsty? Your hypothalamus controls your thirst, and if you're never thirsty then something is out of balance. You should be thirsty enough to hydrate yourself.

What if you drink lots of water and never feel hydrated? Then you're not getting enough electrolytes. Coconut water is a great source of electrolytes, especially good if you're sweating a lot on a hot day or by exercising or have lost a lot of fluids through diarrhea or vomiting.

You can help your cells hydrate by taking the salt test.

Measure out two teaspoons of sea salt and put it in a finger bowl. Drink a big glass of water first thing in the morning and eat a little sea salt. You'll probably find that you crave the salt. During the day keep eating a little sea salt and drinking water until you can't stand anymore salt. At the end of the day measure how much salt is left. Two teaspoons minus whatever was left is how much salt you need to add to your diet. Natural sea salt is rich in minerals. This assumes that you're not eating SAD – the Standard American Diet – which is high in sodium from all the processed foods.

What about other liquids? They don't count. I'm not saying you can't have coffee or tea, but for each cup of caffeinated beverage you must consume a cup of water. Herb teas are fine as long as they are not diuretic – make you urinate – like uva ursi.

And forget sodas. They don't count as hydration. While naturally carbonated mineral water is great for cellular rehydration, the artificial carbonation in soda pop robs your bones of calcium. Plus, soda has too much sugar.

What about diet sodas? First of all, artificial sweeteners cause a surge in insulin. Too much insulin means you're going to lay down more body fat. So they're not really diet, are they? Second, artificial sweeteners are just that – artificial. If nature doesn't make it, you'd better not eat it.

What about natural non-caloric sweeteners like stevia? Stevia is a better choice, but do you know why you prefer sweetened beverages?

There's a study on the sweet perception of diabetics versus people with normal insulin sensitivity. The researchers put different amounts of sugar in a glass of water. Those with healthy insulin sensitivity could perceive the tiniest amount of sugar in the water. It took more than two teaspoons of sugar before diabetics could perceive the sweet taste.

Once you become sensitive to insulin, you won't need to sweeten things.

I start my day by taking my Genesis Gold® first thing in the morning with a big glass of water. Genesis Gold® is a powder. Remember, I first designed it for children to be mixed in juice or applesauce or yoghurt. I have not encapsulated it. Why? Because it's better absorbed as a liquid. When you mix Genesis Gold® with water, it activates the ingredients. The natural ingredients become alive, ready to be absorbed immediately and begin their healing work.

Genesis Gold® naturally hydrates your cells. Take Mary, for instance.

Since Mary went through menopause, she couldn't wear her contacts. After two months of taking Genesis Gold®, her eyes were no longer dry so she began wearing her contacts again. Her optometrist was shocked. Mary's eyes had returned to their natural curvature.

Your eyes are not just the window to your soul. Your eyes reflect the health of your cells.

What about coffee?

After taking my Genesis Gold®, I sit down with a hot beverage, usually a cup of fresh brewed coffee. Full of antioxidants, freshly brewed coffee, like tea, is really good for you. Now, if you drink a pot a day or you have to sweeten it, then it's not so good for you. Studies have shown that coffee drinkers have lower risk of many inflammatory diseases than non-coffee drinkers.

What about alcohol?

It's not a beverage. It's medicinal sugar. It doesn't replace water. That being said, I drink alcohol. I'm Italian. I love red wine. I find especially when I eat red meat, a glass of red wine helps me digest it. Wine is full of antioxidants. And again, studies show that people who drink a moderate amount of alcohol have less inflammatory diseases than nondrinkers.

Everything in moderation.

If you're using alcohol as a drug, then it's no longer good for you. Just like using caffeine for energy or sedating yourself with sugar. Anything you abuse will eventually hurt you.

CHAPTER 12

TOOLS FOR YOUR JOYOUS TRANSFORMATION

I believe achieving your optimal health can be a Joyous Transformation. So now that you've learned all about your amazing body and why it's so very important to balance your Hypothalamus to keep your Hormones in Harmony®, you're probably wondering what more you can do to optimize your health.

Here's more of my best tips to transform yourself – body, mind, and soul.

GET ACTIVE!

If you're going to be healthy, you must be active. The gift of technology is that we don't have to work so hard. The price of technology is our health is declining. Most modern jobs require long hours of sitting on our butts. That's a recipe for insulin resistance, heart disease, and obesity. I don't care what you do, you've got to move.

Dance, run, walk, row, swim, hike, ride a bike. Just move! Every day, do something! And it's best to go outside and get some natural light.

Studies show that insulin resistance increases the more sedentary you are. Get active and get healthy. We spend too much time sitting at work, school, commuting, playing in front of screens rather than getting outside to play. Just 20 minutes of aerobic activity a few days a week will improve insulin sensitivity.

Your metabolism is lowest at night. By sleeping in the dark, high melatonin levels will help reverse insulin resistance. You will begin to notice that you wake up hungry in the morning. That means your adrenal function is normalizing and your hypothalamus is waking up and demanding glucose (the only form of energy the brain uses). So feed it! Start with fruit. After your Genesis Gold®, of course.

Your morning exercise should be aerobic, use interval training to keep your heart rate up. That will set your metabolism at a higher rate for the rest of the day. But if you work out at this pace in the late afternoon, you will have trouble sleeping.

Activity is key in increasing metabolism. Your exercise tolerance and endurance should increase as your hypothalamus balances. In order to burn fat, you must do long slow distances...meaning exercising at a lower heart rate about 60% of your max over 50 minutes to mobilize fat stores. That's because you have 400 calories of glycogen stored in your muscles and liver that must be utilized before your body will burn the triple sugars (triglycerides) stored in your fat cells.

Don't overdo exercise – aerobic activity for 20-30 minutes, 3-5 times a week. Long, slow distances at least once a week. Take one full day off every 5-7 days to allow your hypothalamus to adjust to your new metabolic rate.

Remember, everything in moderation, including exercise. When you exercise, your hypothalamus thinks you're either being chased or chasing something. That's fine for short bursts. But you can overdo it and produce so much cortisol that you break down what you're trying to build up – muscle, bone and cardio-respiratory function. That's not good. That's why you need rest days to strengthen your body.

Before Genesis Gold®, I exercised too much – way, way too much. Miles and miles of running, swimming, and cycling. I would bike to work 50 miles round trip just to fit in more exercise. Nothing was ever enough so I started competing in triathlons. Yes, I was really fit and very lean, but my body was under constant stress. Exercise was my obsession.

Within a month of taking Genesis Gold®, my body said, No More! Oh, I could walk, hike, dance, even run around playing with the kids, but if I put on my heart rate monitor with the intention to go on a long run or ride, my body would balk. My Achilles' tendon would hurt so badly that I could barely walk.

So I was forced to listen to my body. I was afraid I would lose my fitness level, I would get fat, I would go crazy. You see, all those miles and miles of running and cycling kept me sane. I was addicted to the endorphins produced by the runners' high. And like any addiction, I had to go farther and faster to get the high. Too much time exercising, not enough time playing, relaxing, hanging out with my family. It wasn't healthy.

So my body said No and I listened. I hung up my road bike, put away my running shoes, and climbed trees with my kids, rode my horse, danced to my favorite music. Not for hours and hours a day – only short bursts, sort of like how kids and dogs play. I followed their lead and ran around and played outside.

And guess what? I didn't get fat. I didn't go crazy. With Genesis Gold®, my metabolism hummed, my brain function balanced, and I learned to trust my body's innate wisdom. And one year later, my husband asked if I would do a biathlon with him. He would run and I would cycle the same 50 kilometer competition I competed by myself for years. I agreed. So he got down my road bike and cleaned it up. I hadn't been on it for over a year.

That was the best bike ride ever. Without the pressure to compete, I actually enjoyed the scenic course along the coast. And I was only a few minutes off my fastest time. I was shocked. With no training, I was still as fit as ever. I actually could trust my body.

It doesn't matter what you do. Just get active. Get outside. Enjoy nature. And move your body.

If you're short on time, I designed a simple HIT program that takes less than an hour a week to get fit, lean, and reverse insulin resistance. HIT stands for high intensity training.

A cardiovascular surgeon in the United Kingdom wanted to know what was the minimal amount of aerobic activity to improve cardiovascular function, pulmonary function, reverse insulin resistance, increase lean body mass, and decrease body fat. He found it only took three minutes of intense aerobic exercise a week to accomplish all of this.

So I designed a HIT program after his research and challenged a dozen of my patients to try it.

They were all overweight, middle-aged women. Half of them just did the HIT exercises. The other half combined the HIT exercises with my Insulin Resistant Diet.

After six weeks, all of the women had lost body fat, but those following my Insulin Resistant Diet lost the most. Now some of the smaller women did not lose any weight, they lost inches. They went down a whole pant size. I was glad because menopausal and perimenopausal women can't afford to lose lean body mass. We don't want to lose bone or muscle, just that extra padding of fat.

I joined them to see if it was doable. Easy to do and highly effective, I noticed more lean body mass in the first couple of weeks. And my body said Yes!

You can download my HIT exercise at www.thehormonequeen.com/gifts.

Exercise is like a three-legged stool. One leg is strength; one is endurance, and one is flexibility. If you forget any one of these legs, your exercise program is going to fail. Your body needs activity to maintain strength, endurance, and flexibility.

You don't need weights to increase your strength. Use your own body as weight resistance. Yoga and Pilates are great examples of using your body weight to build strength.

Remember to stretch every day. Look at your cat or dog. What does it do when it gets up? It stretches! Why do you think they call that yoga pose "down dog"? Most injuries sustained during exercise are due to lack of flexibility. Your muscles, tendons, and ligaments are too tight and out of balance. As you age, the first thing to go is flexibility. So be kind to yourself and gently stretch your lovely body.

And don't forget to have fun!

SLEEP IN THE DARK

It doesn't matter how well you eat. It doesn't matter how much you exercise.

If you don't get enough sleep, you will get sick. If you don't sleep in the dark, you will stay sick.

Your hormones will not come into balance unless you sleep in the dark. Your brain chemistry will not be balanced unless your sleep in the dark. Your immune system will not protect you and, in fact, may begin to attack you, unless you sleep in the dark. Your gut won't heal unless you sleep in the dark. Nothing will heal unless you sleep in the dark.

Why do you think most critically ill patients do not get better until after they're discharged from the hospital? Because hospitals provide 24/7 care, nurses need light to tend to your needs around the clock. Modern medicine does not get this simple fact. The patient cannot heal completely unless she gets enough sleep in the dark.

If you do nothing else:

- After dark, don't watch TV or do computer work or play on your phone.
- If you absolutely must expose yourself to digital screens after dusk, then wear pink glasses.
- Turn off all light in your bedroom.
- Wake up with the sun.

TAKE TIME TO MEDITATE

Meditation, prayer, time to reflect – whatever you call it – health is not just physical. For optimal health, you must take care of your body, mind, and soul.

Meditation has been shown to lower stress hormones. Meditation is great for hypertension and heart disease. Meditation improves athletic performance. Your body needs you to connect to your soul.

The purpose of meditation is to quiet the mind, to connect to the divine.

You don't have to be sitting still to meditate. You can take meditative walks. Swimming can be meditative. Sweeping can be meditative. Anything done with mindful repetition can be meditative.

When I first opened my integrative health clinic, I had a lot of spiritual gurus going through menopause seek my care. What I mean by spiritual gurus is that they were highly adept psycho-spiritual healers. Physically, they needed help. At the time I hadn't come out of the closet, in terms of admitting my intuitive healing abilities.

One I chose to barter with. We agreed: I would get her hormones balanced and she would teach me to meditate. Sitting before her cross-legged with my hands on my knees, thumbs touching forefingers in the ok sign, I closed my eyes and waited. She just laughed. "This is not your way. Go for a run with that black dog of yours." I hadn't told her about my animals but she was psychic.

So I took her advice and went on a run. Not a mile down the trail and my dog just stopped. She jumped onto a big boulder and stared down at me until I climbed up to join her and sat down. Then she curled up against my back and I closed my eyes, took a few deep breaths, and a purple drop appeared and slowly flooded my consciousness. I was so enchanted by the purple drop that my mind stilled. Soon I was receiving answers to whatever was concerning me.

For years, I found being in nature brought me comfort and insight. It would take a hike, a run, or a swim to find that sweet spot to clear my mind and receive divine guidance. Now it just takes intention.

One meditation I particularly love is more of visualization. I use it to ground myself before doing healing work. A lot of healers, whether conventional or alternative, use their own energy to heal, and eventually they get sick. Most healers have to work on taking care of themselves. I don't believe in using my own energy to heal others but tapping into the universal healing energies.

I begin by standing on the earth, preferably barefoot. But you can stand anywhere with shoes on as long as you're conscious of connecting to the earth. With my feet spaced as wide as my hips, I hold my hands fingertips touching and pointing down against my body, arms relaxed, and breathe. This position makes me feel more open to receive, like my body is a chalice ready to be filled up with divine light.

I imagine the soles of my feet are kissing the earth. I imagine the energy at the level of my hands near my root chakra to be a red glow. I drop that energy like roots down my legs through the soles of my feet and into the earth. I imagine those deep red roots sinking down through the crust of the earth and all the way to the center where I anchor myself. I then allow the energy of the earth to flow back up through those roots and into my body.

As the energy rises, it shifts from red to orange at my belly button and then golden yellow at the level of my diaphragm. I then take a deep breath and imagine the crown of my head is opening like a camera aperture allowing energy to flow in. Violet energy pours into my crown chakra turning indigo blue at the level of my third eye, then bright sky blue at the level of my throat.

Then I imagine the warm earth energies – red, orange, yellow – merge with the cool heavenly energies – violet, indigo, blue – in my heart. The deep forest green of my heart chakra blends with all the colors of the rainbow energies from heaven and earth. I allow the merged energy to flow from my heart to my hands.

Then I place my hands on whatever needs healing – a sore knee, a headache, a broken heart. I am an instrument of healing. It's not my energy but divine energy that does the healing. Plus, I'm never sucked dry when I tap into our beautiful healing earth and the multidimensional heavenly energies.

You can download my guided meditation at
www.thehormonequeen.com/gifts

Taking care of myself – body, mind, and soul – is crucial to my health. And how can I expect my patients to take care of themselves if I don't practice what I preach?

Our bodies are the perfect vehicle for our spiritual transformation. Take good care of yours.

LOVE YOUR BODY

Many of us do not love our bodies. We see ourselves through the dark glasses of self-judgment. A disordered body image leads to eating disorders – maybe not the classic anorexia, but rigid adherence to diets and obsessive exercising. Nor the classic bulimia, but overeating, binge eating, emotional eating. Food becomes the enemy.

I know this to be true for, you see, I was anorexic as a teen. No one knew what anorexia was back then. Karen Carpenter hadn't died from the disease yet. The summer between junior high and high school, I lost 20 pounds. I was never overweight. My parents were horrified. Our family doctor told them to just feed me. The force feedings led to bulimarexia. It wasn't good.

My eating disorder was the beginning of years of being Hormonally Challenged. It's a wonder I ever became pregnant. Between the bulimia and the obsessive exercise, my body fat was so low, I didn't get periods without using hormones.

By 37, I was using bio-identical botanically derived estrogen and progesterone along with lots of supplements. When I began researching Genesis Gold® in 2000, I took myself off everything – hormones and supplements – and joined my 50 plus research subjects.

Within two months, I gained five pounds, my hair and skin improved in texture and moisture, and I got my first un-induced menses. Apparently, I needed that extra weight to make healthy hormones. I've had normal cycles until I became menopausal years later than my younger sisters. Same genetics, same Mediterranean diet, similar stress exposures. The only difference – I'm taking Genesis Gold®.

Yet the greatest change was the healing of my body image. I began to appreciate my body. It was strong. It was fit. It was in pretty darn good shape for having two kids. After years of amenorrhea, I appreciated my periods. My mother and grandmother had no appreciation for their menses. It was more of a nuisance than a blessing. The women in my family had lovely figures but they hated their bodies and it was passed down through the generations.

I was determined not to pass on this curse of body hatred to my daughter. So I began treating myself extra special during that time of the month. So special, that my prepubescent daughter couldn't wait to get her period. By the time Kyra became a young woman and took delight in her beautiful healthy body, I felt like the curse had been broken.

Slowly over the years, I fell in love with my body.

Those who've been sober for many years will still refer to themselves as alcoholics. Once you have an eating disorder, you tend to have a disordered body image. You may not be actively anorexic, bulimic, or overeating, yet you still look at yourself with those same eyes. As I came into harmony with myself, my eating disorder released its hold on my mindset. I began to see it as a maladaptive coping mechanism, like smoking, and found other healthier ways to de-stress. Because frankly, just like any addiction, bulimia was my way of dealing with fear.

Healing my disordered body image was one of the greatest gifts I received from Genesis Gold®.

Truth be told, I have had few patients who have not benefited from consuming Genesis Gold®. I have treated multiple endocrine disorders, neurological disorders and immune disorders since Genesis Gold® has been available, and the majority of my patients have been able to get off their other supplements, hormone replacement therapies, and medications.

I believe if you feed the body what it needs, it will heal.

My healing vibration is within everything I create – especially Genesis Gold®. I feed it to my animals who outlive their natural life spans, and many of my patients have used Genesis Gold® with their pets as well. No belief systems there, just healing.

We are genetically encoded for perfect health. Dis-ease is maladaptive genetics turned on by poor dietary and lifestyle choices.

Genesis Gold® is designed in golden means proportions to upregulate genetic potential, optimizing health and vitality.

THE MOST HORMONALLY CHALLENGED OF ALL

Elizabeth was thirty-something when she came to me. She had been diagnosed with hypopanpituitarism – she made none of her own hormones. No adrenal hormones, no thyroid hormones, no sex hormones. She wanted bio-identical hormone replacement rather than the synthetics she had been taking for years. She had never had a period and only with obsessive exercise and hormone replacement therapy was she able to keep her weight under control.

She did very well on the bio-identicals for years. When I finally got Genesis Gold® manufactured, she agreed to give it a try. Over the next eighteen months, she was able to wean off her hormones, all of them, and had her own periods. I told her it was time to think about contraception. She laughed. She still believed what the doctors had told her all her life – she was infertile.

At the age of 43, Elizabeth gave birth to a healthy baby boy. She has been off hormones ever since. I suspect that when she gets close to menopause, she may need some transitional bio-identical hormone supplementation.

Elizabeth is my most dramatic case. I have had lots of other patients with hypothalamic dysfunction who have been able to start functioning on their own with Genesis Gold®.

You don't have to be as out of balance as Elizabeth to benefit from taking Genesis Gold®.

HEALING TAKES TIME

Your current state of health did not happen overnight. Who you are now is a result of years of choices. Lifestyle choices including what you eat, when you sleep, how much activity you get, what toxins you've been exposed to, even your belief systems affect your health.

Choosing to take Genesis Gold® is making a commitment to your future health. For those newly ill, most recently out of balance, it may take weeks or months to optimize their health. For those out of balance for many years, it'll take longer.

It's like making the choice to quit smoking. Let's say you've smoked a pack a day since you were a teenager, then you quit. You feel worse before you feel better. You cough up pretty yucky stuff as your lungs clear out years of toxicity. If you've smoked for 30 years, it takes at least 30 months to restore healthy lung function.

Same with Genesis Gold®. Most people find it when their health is truly challenged. Oftentimes they've tried many therapies before finding my website, reading an article, or being referred by a friend. I counsel them that according to how long they've been ill is reflected by how long it'll take to restore wellness.

Those who commit to taking Genesis Gold® as their daily foundational support will keep optimizing their health.

Genesis Gold® has adaptogenic herbs to help support your adrenals, sea vegetation to support your thyroid, whole plant nutrients to optimize digestion, detoxification, immunity, energy production and balance your sex hormones as well as the Sacred Seven® amino acids to balance your hypothalamus. Genesis Gold® provides foundational support for lasting change.

You can find Genesis Gold® at
www.thehormonequeen.com/genesisgold

Remember – Balance comes with Time.

CHAPTER 13

YOU'VE GOT THE POWER

Rubber gloves blown up to resemble chickens float across the floor of the exam room. After reading all the books we brought, we're now drawing on the exam table paper. We've been waiting over an hour and a half and the doctor has not shown up. It's all I can do to entertain my child.

For a kindergartener, Jarys is exceedingly patient. Not me. I'm fit to be tied that we have to be evaluated by an adult endocrinologist from our HMO. The insurance company wants to switch Jarys' growth hormone injections to a cheaper version. My intuition says this is a bad idea. Switching hormones can have dire effects. Insulin dependent diabetics can't be switched from porcine-derived insulin to bovine-derived insulin and then go back. They develop antibodies. And then what? Nothing works. I'm not going to take that chance with Jarys.

Gruffly opening the door, the doctor bursts in. "It looks like this kid needs Ritalin, not growth hormone."

I gather Jarys into my arms and say over his head, "If you were qualified to evaluate pediatric patients, your exam rooms would be set up for their needs. We made the best of the ridiculous amount of time you made a five-year-old wait."

The doctor kicks aside the chicken balloons and sits down. "You realize that he's cost this clinic over two million dollars."

That's it! I pick Jarys up, and sit him on the edge of the exam table, before turning to face the doctor. Jarys wraps his little arms around my neck and starts to cry. The mother bear in me erupts, "If this HMO clinic had provided the proper obstetric care, we would not be here now!"

An HMO was the only option offered by the city my husband worked for. At the time, we had no other insurance choice. HMOs gamble on signing up the young and healthy. With ample premiums coming in, they provide bulk monthly checks to doctors to care for the masses, banking on the fact that these healthy patients rarely seek care. Unfortunately for us and the system, our child was born needing much more care.

Before the doctor can defend his position, I add, "I've done the research. We're not switching growth hormone to save a few dollars. The protropin's working."

Thankfully, I won that insurance battle and many others over the years. Because of Jarys' preexisting health issues, no other insurance would take us, especially when his growth hormone injections cost over $3000 a month.

As a health care provider, I chose not to work for HMOs. I wanted to be paid for the health care services I provided my patients, not better compensated for not delivering care.

When I first graduated UCLA as a neophyte Nurse Practitioner, I worked for an urgent care. That's where I got my first taste of HMOs from the provider's point of view. Working alongside physicians, I was surprised when they would check the insurance coverage of a patient before seeing them. Most of the time, they passed the HMO patients on to me, preferring to see PPO patients for higher compensation. Plus, they received monthly stipends for their HMO patients. They were adamant that I not do "too much testing". Anything beyond basic care for these HMO patients was taken out of their monthly stipends and cost the clinic.

My experiences with HMOs, both as a patient and a provider, was a two-part gift.

First, I developed my medical detective skills by honing my assessment and examination skills without relying on diagnostic testing. I got really good at what the docs called vet medicine. I learned to rely on my intuition to guide me, so when I did order diagnostic tests, the results were profoundly significant. The specialists I would refer my patients to started to take notice of my diagnostic skills.

I was surprised that my colleagues could not feel what was so evident to me. One general surgeon would take my referrals in spite of negative imaging tests, asking only for diagnostic coding to cover the surgery, for case after case, he would open the patient up and find exactly what I described.

I would place my hands on a patient and their tumors were so obvious, I thought the other doctors were not examining the patients thoroughly enough. I can smell disease, see anatomical anomalies, hear murmurs. My collaborating physician explained that providers with a musical ear were more likely to hear murmurs. I didn't think I had a musical ear.

I know now that my "skills" are more vibrational. I feel the energy of disease and my senses pick it up. I often dream of a patient before meeting them. When they arrive in my office, I already know what's wrong. I already examined them in my dreams.

I can also feel the psycho-emotional roots of their ailments. They may be complaining of some ache or pain, but as they describe the bothersome symptom, I perceive something deeper. Something happened in their life that created the ailment. For me, it's like watching a movie montage. Images of events flash before my mind's eye, and using my medical detective skills, I make the connection. The patients are always surprised that I know what I know. I'm not. I got my medical intuitive gifts honestly. Both my grandmother and my mother had it. They just didn't have the scientific language and medical training to make sense of what they were perceiving. I do.

The second gift of my early exposure to HMOs, both as a patient and a provider, was that it became the foundation for starting my own fee-for-service practice – Full Circle Family Health.

FULL CIRCLE FAMILY HEALTH

In July 1997, I left a conventional medical practice and started my own integrative health care practice – Full Circle Family Health. Since I believe if you heal the woman, she heals her family, my female patients got better and began bringing their spouses and children, parents and siblings, friends and coworkers to see me. Truly family health care.

Before starting my private practice, I sought my mother's advice as a small business owner. She thought I was crazy wanting to be an entrepreneur. "It's not easy, Deb. You won't make the money you did as an employee. You won't get paid vacations. You'll have to worry about taxes and bills, licenses and insurance. You'll have to pay your staff and all your bills before paying yourself."

Mom was right. But what I did get is the freedom to provide health care in a way that truly helps my patients. Because right off the bat, I chose not to take health insurance. Patients paid out of their pocket to see me and then submitted to their own insurance company for reimbursement. One-third of my patients from the conventional medical practice didn't have insurance and paid cash to see me – not the doctor I worked for, but me. So I was pretty sure this cash-based business would work. Plus, I refused to be tied down by insurance companies trying to tell me how to practice. And in the end, their reimbursement rate per hour was less than I was paying my assistant.

I asked Mom to run my practice. At first, she balked. "I don't know anything about health care." No, but she knew lots about running a small business. She ran a copy shop for two decades, putting my sisters and me through college, and making money even after Kinkos moved to town. She knew lots about customer service, and that's what I believe was missing in the health care system.

You see, the customer is the one who pays for your services. In the health care system, insurance is the one who directly reimburses the doctors, the clinics, the hospitals. Insurance companies are catered to like customers, not the patients.

And I noticed over the years that patients who paid out of their pocket were much more motivated to take care of themselves, much more likely to incorporate the health education I was providing into their lives, much more likely to get better. The less the patients paid directly to the health care provider, the less motivated they were to do the work necessary to heal. It's as if they assumed they had gotten ten-dollar care for their ten-dollar copay. And we are a money driven society. We place a higher value on products and services that cost more.

So I don't accept insurance. And I have highly motivated patients who are willing to do what it takes to get better.

Most of my patients do have insurance. They just pay out of their pocket to see me. They also pay out of their pocket for other complementary healers like acupuncturists. They believe their health is worth the cost. And at Full Circle Family Health, they get what they pay for.

Rather than medicate, I educate my patients. Poor things come so Hormonally Challenged that they cannot possibly absorb all I have to teach them. Yet there are no stupid questions. I teach them, coach them, cheerlead them. I partner with my patients to help them achieve optimal health.

If I had a dime for every time a patient said "How come no one else could figure out my problem?" I would be able to retire. I figure out the roots of their dis-ease because I listen to them. I am willing to go where other providers fear to venture. I investigate alternatives and am willing to try new things with my patients. I've always pushed the envelope and have found that I am five to seven years ahead of current thinking, current procedure, current practice.

Most doctors and nurse practitioners are caring healers but few have been trained in the art of balancing hormones, let alone the entire neuro-immune-endocrine system. I have been honing my craft for a long time. It's not easy for most providers to get a feel for hormones. Just as each prescription is individually prepared by a compounding pharmacist, it requires an in-depth consult to individualize the therapy for each patient.

When I first opened Full Circle Family Health, one of the local gynecological surgeons called me.

"Deborah, I'm sending you all my weird hormone patients."

I thanked him and asked what was so "weird" about them.

"Well, in medical school," he answered, "you learn that A leads to B and occasionally C, but I get to Z and still can't figure out these weird hormone cases."

"That's because, Dr. G," I explained, "endocrinology is not an exact science. It's an art."

"I'm a surgeon" he sighed. "and since you're the artist, you can take care of them."

That's when I came up with the term "Hormonally Challenged." Health care providers are as challenged by hormonal issues as their patients.

So I blend the art of healing with the science of medicine to help my Hormonally Challenged patients. In the first consult, I spend two hours:

- Gathering information regarding the history of their symptoms, their family history, their lifestyle, their sex life, their spiritual life.

- Spend time explaining how their body works specifically in regards to their concerns.

- Explore factors that may influence their neuro-immune-endocrine health like nutritional deficiencies, environmental toxicities, sleep patterns, immune function, life stressors, relationships (intimate, dependent, and professional), disordered eating and body image, and their beliefs about healing.

- Do a complete physical exam, taking time to educate them about their body and how to take care of it – like how to perform self-breast and self-testicular exams. Most patients learn more about their bodies in that two hours than in a lifetime living in it.

- Assess adrenal and thyroid disorders, insulin resistance, immune dysfunction, neurological and mood disorders, intestinal malabsorption, detoxification issues as well as other major health problems.

- Order the appropriate lab tests for them.

- Do appropriate psycho-spiritual counseling – if they are open to receive it – which most are now that I'm open to receive them.

- Design a healing protocol specifically for them including therapeutic nutrition, lifestyle changes, and psycho-spiritual homework.

STRIVING FOR SYMBIOTIC HEALTH CARE

In biology, we learn that there are two types of relationships – symbiotic and parasitic.

An example of a symbiotic relationship is your beneficial gut bacteria. You house them and feed them. In return, they help you digest your food, activate the micronutrients in your food, and protect you from invasion.

A parasitic relationship is like a yeast infection. Overgrowth of Candida in your mouth, your intestines, your vagina causes inflammation. The yeast is feeding off you and giving nothing back. That's parasitic.

We have symbiotic and parasitic relationships with others. Symbiosis is when you partner with another person and both use your talents equally to achieve a goal. You know you're in a parasitic relationship with another person when you feel sucked dry, you're giving more than you're receiving, or vice versa, you're taking more than you're giving. It's not good for either of you.

Our current health care system is parasitic. It feeds off dis-ease.

Insurance pays poorly or not at all for health education to empower patients. It pays by diagnosis. The more dis-eased, the more it pays. Yet you cannot treat everything at once.

No, insurances do not pay well if you try to take care of all the patient's concerns in one visit. It pays to have the patient come back again and again for each complaint.

And there is no time to educate, let alone empower the patient.

Our health care system encourages parasitic relationships between health care providers and patients. If you get them well, you lose money.

I once worked for a doctor who complained that I gave the patients too much information. He said: "If they know too much, they won't need us."

I left his parasitic practice and opened my own – a symbiotic health care practice. Free from the confines of insurance reimbursement, I am able to spend time educating my patients. And they get better. And then they send their friends and family. I never advertise. My whole practice is word of mouth referrals.

I insist on symbiotic relationships with my patients. We are partners in their health care. I educate rather than medicate. I try to shine the light of illumination on their dis-ease – how their lifestyle choices, environmental influences, and belief systems affect their physiology, what maladaptive genes might be lurking in their DNA and how to change their genetic expression. Yes, it is possible to transform DNA – it's why I created Genesis Gold®.

I've found that Genesis Gold® often brings our parasitic relationships up to the surface of our consciousness. I created Genesis Gold® to heal maladaptive genetic expression, one of which is vulnerability to parasites. Our body mirrors our soul lessons. Genesis Gold® illuminates that which no longer serves, so we might release it.

As my patients take more responsibility, own their past choices and begin to transform their lives, they experience gnosis – they "know" innately in their bodies the truth of their dis-ease and begin to heal.

TIPS FOR PARTNERING WITH YOUR HEALTH CARE PROVIDER

- Adopt a partnership attitude. They are not GOD and you are not a victim.

- Be responsible for your health. While you are paying them for their medical expertise, remember you can heal yourself.

- Ask questions and expect answers.

- Do your homework so you know your options.

- Decide on what recommendations you are willing to follow and report the results.

- If you cannot complete a prescribed course of treatment, tell them why.

- Have a positive, hopeful outlook.

- Do NOT make fear-based decisions.

- Remember, thought creates reality. Expect a positive attitude from your health care provider.

- Express your gratitude for your healing ability and their help.

THE CIRCLE OF LIFE

Elijah came to me in the fall of 2002 diagnosed with lung cancer. Since I was a clinical endocrine advisor in a research project using natural progesterone to treat cancer at the Sansum Medical Clinic, Elijah's lawyer, also a patient of mine, thought I could help.

Cancer is not my specialty, yet miscommunication in the neuro-immune-endocrine system is at the root of most dis-ease. So I spent two hours going over Elijah's history, looking for signs of age-related decline that could be at the root of his illness, trying to understand why this brilliant man's body was failing him at 52, and explaining the biochemistry of cancer as related to the complicated system of hormonal miscommunication with DNA.

I drew this out for Elijah:

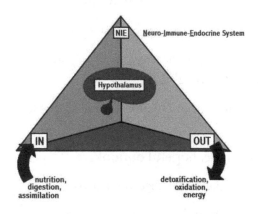

Excitedly Elijah asked, "So you have something to balance my ligands?"

Ligands are molecules that bind to cell receptor sites. Hormones and neurotransmitters act as ligands.

Elijah was brilliant, one of the only patients who understood the scientific lingo of my theories. He was even open to the psycho-spiritual roots of dis-ease, including the irony of being afflicted with cancer after inventing thermal implants to treat brain tumors.

Elijah knew that if we could balance the ligands of his neuro-immune-endocrine system we could possibly reverse the genetic mutations that caused his cancer.

In fact, I did have something for him – my Genesis Gold® formula to balance the hypothalamic orchestration of the neuro-immune-endocrine system, but in theory only. After completing pilot studies the year before, my personal funds ran out and I struggled to find a manufacturer to mix even a small batch. Elijah took my hand and offered to help.

"No," I protested, "you came here for me to help you."

"Perhaps I came to help you. My cancer was a fortuitous portal for our meeting."

Thus began our journey to manufacture my formula so he might partake of it. Elijah truly believed he would be cured by my invention.

In the meantime, I recommended a natural treatment regime, since he was opposed to traditional therapies, and spent much time counseling him. He treated me as a beloved daughter, introducing me to colleagues who would forge the path to the birth of my nutraceutical product. Becoming attached, I searched for cures for his cancer.

The day I brought the first bottle of Genesis Gold® to him, Elijah smiled, beckoned me closer and whispered, "I knew you could do it."

It was his last lucid moment. At the request of his family, I had been coming to his lovely villa in the hills of Santa Barbara to help him die. As a nurse practitioner, I treated the walking well. Some patients had passed over the years, usually of old age, occasionally untimely, but not since being a neophyte nurse had I witnessed death.

After graduating nursing school in 1983, I worked on a surgical floor at UCLA Medical Center. We saw the sickest of patients – heart transplants, complete surgical resections of the bowels, lung resections. My first encounter with death was a young woman the same age as me dying of pancreatic cancer.

When I arrived on the night shift and saw her Do Not Resuscitate order, I knew her family and physicians had given up. Not me! I wasn't going to let her drown in her own secretions!

I stayed by her bedside suctioning her tracheostomy. Her intern refused to give me a permanent suction order so that I could take care of my other three patients, so I handed him the suction catheter and called the chief resident.

My colleagues were appalled. No one called the chief in the middle of the night, especially not a nurse.

Amazingly, he wasn't upset, but asked if I saw the DNR order. "Dr. Hope, I'm not resuscitating her. I just don't want her to be alone. I..." Seeing the intern escape down the hall, I tried to hang up on the chief.

"Oh, no, you don't. We're going to discuss why you can't let her die." I resisted, but he kept me on the phone until it was too late.

The charge nurse helped me prepare the young woman's body for the morgue. And with tears, I was forced to let my patient go.

Twenty years later, I was not so resistant. Elijah's family left me alone with him. I sat at his bedside and meditated on how I could help him pass. I had already counseled with each of his family members. When I thought of his recalcitrant son who had finally agreed to see his father after our phone conversation that morning, I felt a wave of gratitude. And it wasn't mine, it was from Elijah. I opened my eyes.

His diminished energy, faded to non-existent in his limbs, now concentrated in his heart chakra, shimmered. I gasped to see a funnel of light connect to him. He appeared to lift from his form – pure white light, not the fiery red of his life force – and enter the conical shaped energy. Other light forms greeted him, ancestors and guides, passing him along to the end. And at the infinite end of this brilliant white light was pure Love. He was enveloped, embraced like long lost lovers, the encounter so intimate, I was torn between turning away in deference to such a private moment and watching in awe.

Suddenly, Elijah's essence turned away from the Light and I was swept up to see from his perspective. It appeared as if the room where his body lay, even me at his bedside, existed in a fishbowl. The reality was the Light, the physical existence, an illusion.

We all have a purpose here on earth. Some of us take decades to fulfill our soul purpose, others but a few precious years. As much as I believe death is but transition to a lighter form of consciousness, still it's hard for those left behind to let go of the physical. We are in love with the form. Many of us do not see the soul light in each other when alive, so it's hard to be open to receive them when they pass.

As a Family Nurse Practitioner, I have brought babies into this world and helped the dying release their bodies. Midwifing Elijah through the portal of death was his second gift to me. The experience taught me to be open to receive the gift in every encounter.

Life is a circle. As a healer, I had taken a very long time to release my savior complex, to understand that I was not responsible for my patients' illnesses, nor could I take credit for their cures.

I'm a partner in my patients' healing path, holding the space in which they recover or not – it's always their choice.

THE TIME IS RIPE TO RECEIVE

So why did I wait so long to write this book? I've been doing this healing work since 1997. I published a novel eight years before this book. Why? Because the time is just now ripe. I believe the health care system is ripe for change. You are reading this book now because you are ripe for healing. My patients come to me when they are ripe for healing. And I had to be ripe before sharing this with you.

Everything happens for a reason. We often have to let go in order to receive. Death becomes a birth. Our former selves must die in order for our new self to be born. Menopause feels very much like a death and a birth.

My mom was there when I birthed my first child. My mom helped me birth Full Circle Family Health, then five years later, helped me birth Genesis Gold®. And it was her death that helped me birth this book.

On January 6th, 2015, I took one look at my mother and knew life was about to change. Mom was sick, really sick. And I know sick. I can smell disease, feel tumors, see death. And Mom rarely ever gets sick. But after flying to spend Christmas with one of my sisters in Utah and then driving from LAX to Big Bear to entertain my youngest sister's family for New Year's, Mom was tired. And she's never tired! My mom is the Energizer Bunny! Plus, she had a strange rash on her legs.

So that day, despite being "my worst patient" as she proudly claimed, Mom got up on my exam table so I could check her out.

The rash turned out to be phlebitis and I didn't like what I felt in her stomach. An abdominal ultrasound confirmed my suspicions. So I consulted with my collaborating physician and ordered a CT scan and a venous Doppler. Mom's bloodwork didn't look great either.

The next week, as I was orchestrating Mom's care, one of the twins texted that she was driving from Northern California to check in on

Dad. My parents divorced twenty-five years earlier but still lived in the same town. Mom drove up to Ojai to stay and work with me. And she insisted on driving the seventy miles back home so we could have our separate lives. A very self-sufficient woman, our mother, raised us to be strong and independent, as well.

Dad seemed to have the same neurological symptoms he had five years earlier, so I set up an appointment with his neurosurgeon, ordered blood and an MRI. Mom had a tendency to focus more on others than herself, so I didn't think she needed to know about Dad yet, and she was adamant that I not tell my sisters about her until we knew more.

So the next morning, I'm with Mom at the interventional radiology center getting her liver biopsied while juggling calls from my sister regarding Dad's medical care. When it rains, it pours.

That evening my sisters were giving me a hard time for not getting more involved with Dad. I went in to check on Mom and she took one look at my face and asked, "What's wrong?"

"Please," I begged her, "let me tell my sisters." She agreed.

I called a conference call with my three sisters. "This isn't about Dad. It's about Mom." And then the tears began to flow.

The great weight was lifted for a short time. The next day Mom insisted on going back home to pack. Since her venous Doppler showed no signs of deep vein thrombosis, my collaborating physician and the interventional radiologist agreed that she could go home. I let her go, knowing my sister would stay with her.

But Mom felt fine and sent my sister home!

Early the next morning, I got a call from Mom's partner. "Deb, the paramedics are here and they want to speak to you." I instructed the emergency personnel that Mom probably had a pulmonary embolism. By the time I got to the ER in her home town, they had brought her back to life three times.

I walked into the emergency room, the same one I volunteered as a candy striper before going to UCLA nursing school in 1981. There I found my mom intubated, panicking, but very much alive. I kissed her, tried to orient her, asked the nurse to please sedate her, and consulted with the emergency physicians. Then I texted my sisters. "You need to come now." They all flew in that evening. By then, Mom was in the ICU.

This was Mom's worse nightmare. I know nearly dying, being intubated and tied down (yes, they use soft restraints to keep patients from pulling out their ventilation tube) would be most people's worst nightmare – but being taken to that particular hospital was hers. You see, both her parents died in that hospital.

In December 1982, my beloved grandparents moved from Philadelphia to California to be near their only daughter and granddaughters. I was just a nursing student at UCLA, but when Poppop got off that plane, I knew he was going to die. And he did, three weeks later. And less than two years later, Nana died in that same hospital. Mom never ever wanted to go there...but there she was in the ICU, unable to communicate with a tube down her throat and her hands tied down. Have you ever seen anyone yell with their eyes?

Thank goodness for my daughter Kyra, a tele/ICU nurse, who knew those machines like the back of her hand. The rest of us nurses...yes, three out of four daughters...hadn't been practicing in the hospital for years.

Five days after that fatalistic call, Mom was discharged from the hospital into my care. She had terminal stage IV cancer. They gave her a couple of months. I gave her more. She wasn't ready to go quite yet. She told me that her cancer would change everything for me.

Mom was right. Everything changed.

I had to take over her job at managing the business – all three – Full Circle Family Health, Genesis Health Products, and Divine Daughters Unite, the charity she founded with me in 2007. I told you Mom was the Energizer Bunny! She managed all this and made time for all nine of her grandchildren, her two great grandchildren and of course, her four daughters. She had never been sick a day in her life and felt blessed to have outlived her parents by a dozen years.

So I kept our heads above water while trying desperately to help Mom. She wasn't going for conventional treatment – she didn't believe in it. Besides the oncologists had very little to offer for her advanced cancer. By the end of April, I got her healthy enough to spend time with my sisters and her grandchildren. By June, she had made it to my youngest sister. Five weeks later, I flew to Texas to get her into hospice care.

On July 21st, I held my mother in my arms as she took her last breath.

We all miss her terribly. Mom was a bright light for so many. She loved working at Full Circle Family Health – it fulfilled her dream. She always wanted to be a nurse. She birthed three nurses and one grand-nurse, but never went back to school to fulfill her own dream. Mom was very, very intuitive. She was kind of like having a human CT scanner in the office. She felt things. I got my intuitive gifts from her.

My patients adored her. One told me she still hears Mom's voice when she falls off her healing program. "Why don't you love yourself enough to take care of you?"

The day Mom died, I had just finished releasing hospice, calling all the relatives, comforting my family, when I got a call from a financial institution. I wasn't going to take it, but I felt Mom push me.

"Congratulations, you got the business credit line!"

I couldn't believe it. Mom and I had tried for the past five years to get enough funding for Genesis Health Products to grow and no one would take a chance on us.

"Thanks, Mom!"

"Ma'am, my name is Todd."

"I'm not thanking you, Todd. I'm thanking my Mom. She's already pulling strings from heaven!"

Todd didn't get it, but I did.

Mom was helping me birth once again. Finally, a manufacturer who could keep us supplied with Genesis Gold® showed up (thanks,

Mom!). Then a publisher for this book (thanks again, Mom!). And when I finally sat down to write it, guess who became my muse?

Every time I got stuck, Mom came to me. In dreams and visions, sometimes I heard her voice reminding me of how our healing journey began. When I got so focused on writing about hormones, my iPad blanked out. We were camping at the time, so there was no other computer available. I lay on the beach wondering why and I heard Mom's voice: *Don't forget the children.* And I was in our old office kneeling before little Alex – the little boy who spurred my desire to create the "brew" that became Genesis Gold®.

We were always close. As a young child, I felt Mom's emotion. I felt her when she was sick. I felt her all through our lives, through the transforming journey of her cancer, no matter how far away she was. So I am not surprised to still feel her with me even after death.

Mom was right. Her illness changed everything. And her death gave me the courage to share what I know about healing with you. Thanks, Mom!

YOUR HEALING TRANSFORMATION

Everything that happens in our life changes us. How we perceive the events in our lives is how the change ultimately affects us. Most of us live ordinary, unexciting lives, perhaps not feeling fulfilled, but we exist. In super human mode, we do everything for everyone else, losing ourselves in the process. We lose our sense of identity, our self-respect, even our health. Most of us need a crisis event to change our ways and start taking care of ourselves.

Your healing transformation begins when you recognize the need to change.

I truly enjoy working with the Hormonally Challenged. Why? Because the incompetence of our hormones make us ripe for change. Like a ripple in a pond, when you make a healthy transformation, you affect everything and everyone around you. By healing ourselves, we heal our families, our communities, our world.

Most of my middle-age patients find the change granted by menopause or andropause to be a true transformation. Many have gone back to school, started new careers, begun practicing their true craft. I cannot tell you how many professional women I have treated that have become artists at this time of life, not just as a hobby, but making money at expressing themselves in the form of art.

Like a caterpillar, you spend most of your early life going from leaf to leaf wondering when you will be able to fly. At mid-life, you enter the cocoon stage. You pull in all your resources, wrap yourself up, hoping to survive the hormonal rollercoaster. Then by the time you reach the pause, you become a butterfly. Finally, you can fly!

Just like Dorothy in the <u>Wizard of Oz</u>, you've been wearing the ruby slippers the whole time, you just didn't realize it.

It's time to tap into your innate power to heal.

Perhaps your fears and doubts may be creeping up. You may feel unsure of your ability to experience optimal health.

You're not alone. You have this book to help you along your healing journey.

Remember your hormones sing and your DNA dances.

And your Hypothalamus is the maestro of your entire system.

All you have to do is feed your hypothalamus to harmonize your hormones and your DNA will dance optimal health.

That's why I created Genesis Gold® - to support your hypothalamus and optimize your health from the inside out.

Genesis Gold® is like the Yellow Brick Road leading you to discover your innate healing ability.

You can manifest anything. Even change your genetic expression to heal.

You have the power to heal yourself.

APPENDIX

GIFTS FOR YOU

On my website, I set up a special gift page for you to download my diets, recipes, exercise program, and guided meditation.

Just go to: www.thehormonequeen.com/gifts

This is a private page just for you, my reader. Be sure to use the link above or type it in to access the gift page.

Here you will find:

- DMAR® Nutritional Path to Wellness

- My Insulin Resistant Diet

- My Liver Cleanse

- My HIT Exercise

- My Healing Meditation

    You can find more information about Genesis Gold® at:
    www.thehormonequeen.com/genesisgold

If you choose to partake of my gifts, I will send you a special reader's discount on Genesis Gold®.

And for even more Hormone Healing Tips & Advice, please join my Hormone Reboot Training:

http://thehormonequeen.genesisgold.com/hnh-hormone-reboot-training/

Thank you for including me on your healing journey.

Love and Light,

Deborah

ABOUT THE AUTHOR

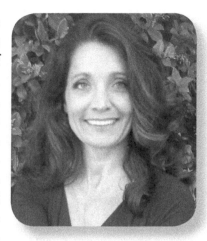

The Hormone Queen® Deborah Maragopoulos MN FNP blends the Science of Medicine with the Art of Healing. Upon graduating from UCLA with a Masters in Nursing, Deborah studied nutritional science, functional medicine, quantum physics, genetics, neuro-immune-endocrinology, and metaphysical healing. Through clinical research and two decades of collecting empirical data Deborah developed a unique holistic health care model blending naturopathic and allopathic therapies, as well as a promising nutraceutical product – Genesis Gold®. Because of her success with the most challenging cases, patients come from around the world to her Intuitive Integrative Health Care practice – Full Circle Family Health. An inspirational speaker, Deborah has shared her pearls of wisdom at the California Women's Expo, the Southern California Women's Herbal Symposium, and the American College of Nurse Practitioners. Her debut novel LoveDance® was awarded Reviewers Choice for Best Spiritual Fiction; its proceeds are donated to Divine Daughters Unite, a nonprofit Deborah created to empower young women through compassionate service. Founder of Genesis Health Products Inc, former clinical endocrine advisor to Genova Laboratory and Sansum Medical Clinic, and past president of California Association of Nurse Practitioners, Deborah lives with her husband in the beautiful Ojai Valley. www.thehormonequeen.com